Reclaiming the Wisdom of the Body

RECLAIMING THE WISDOM OF THE BODY

A Personal Guide to Chinese Medicine

SANDRA HILL

A Citadel Press Book
Published by Carol Publishing Group

CONTENTS

Acknowledgements   vii
Introduction   1
Glossary   9

Part 1
THE PHILOSOPHY OF CHINESE MEDICINE
Understanding the Body   11

Part 2
THE BODILY LANDSCAPE
Learning about Energy Flow   57

Part 3
BALANCING HEAVEN AND EARTH
General Exercises   105

Part 4
WORKING WITH THE FIVE ELEMENTS
Practical Ways to Strengthen Your Particular Weakness   157

Part 5
COMMON IMBALANCES
Practical Remedies for Everyday Problems   201

Conclusion   240
Further Reading   242
Index   243

ACKNOWLEDGEMENTS

I would like to thank all my teachers, particularly Dr Hiroshi Motoyama, Claude Larre SJ and Elisabeth Rochat de la Vallée. A special thankyou to Peter Firebrace for his inspiration and support in our work together, and to Kikan Massara and Mary Parsons for their advice and encouragement.

INTRODUCTION

Within the discipline of Chinese medicine it is easy to get caught up in the theory, in the details of clinical practice, even in the poetry of the ancient texts. It is a vast subject with many schools and traditions. The theory has become so complex, the detail so intricate that we can never know enough. There is always more to learn, more to know. Throughout its long history it has often been in the interest of the few to keep knowledge secret and obscure, and there have been many attempts to make Chinese medicine complex and esoteric. But at its heart it is very simple. It is based on common sense and the careful observation of nature. If something is cold, it needs to be warmed. If there is blockage, it needs to be dispersed. The complexity lies in the ability to observe, to tune in and to listen.

Although I began with the intention of writing this book for my patients, and with the hope that others might find it useful or inspiring, as I have progressed I have realised that I have in fact written it for myself, to get me out of my head and back into my body, away from complexity and detail and back to the simple truths that lie at the heart of Chinese medicine.

It often takes illness for us to slow down, take stock and get back to what's important, even for those of us who should know better. A few years ago I had pneumonia and although I had taken time off and rested, I was still experiencing chest pain quite some time later. I decided to have some checks. The usual tests were run and I was told that there was nothing wrong. For a woman of my age I was pretty healthy. I should consider myself lucky. But the fact that I was in pain was not taken into account as machines printed out figures and X-rays told that all was clear. My subjective experience was invalidated, my body-knowing given no credence at all.

A visit to a Chinese herbalist brought a different kind of dissatisfaction. This time I was listened to but I was given no information, no advice on how to help myself or how to prevent future problems. Yet again I met the caring mask of the expert saying, 'Don't you worry, just leave this to me.' I knew I had pain; I knew all was not well. I had tried most alternatives and no-one else seemed to be able to help. It was time to do those things that I tell people to do every day – such as rest, take time off, look at the deeper implications of the illness.

Real change seems to occur when we begin to take responsibility for our own health, and begin to listen to the messages of the body. This is not easy in a society where we have been encouraged to leave it to the professionals. Our health is an area where many of us readily relinquish responsibility though at the same time feeling a growing sense of unease because we are not heard. Medicine has become so technological, so removed from our feelings, that we have all but forgotten that our bodies are intelligent. Our bodies know how to heal cuts, mend bones, make babies, and our body-knowing can often tell us much that technology will miss. Our refined senses of smell, touch, taste give us constant feedback about the suitability of our environment, our food, our homes, but our rational minds, in love with technology and scientific proof, have learnt not to listen.

After 12 years as a practising acupuncturist I believe that there is little that I can do unless patients are willing to engage actively in their own healing. Maybe I can fix something for a while – take away a symptom here, a symptom there, but both for patient and practitioner I feel that that is no longer enough. A successful acupuncture treatment does not merely relieve symptoms, it helps the patient to understand the problem. This can happen in many ways. As I spend time with my patients I feed back information I am receiving from the pulse, the tongue, the body shape, the body feel, and in the symbolic language of the Chinese medical classics I attempt to create a picture they can work with. This will often involve the concepts of yin and yang, heaven and earth, the five elements, the five spirits, the seven emotions. Explaining what I am doing and why has often proved to be a valuable tool in engaging the patient in the healing process. The imagery is potent and has its own healing power.

While the treatment is in progress, I may encourage the patient to be silent and look within. This is the second important tool of self-healing. During acupuncture treatment many patients describe sensations and feelings, thoughts and insights which are the beginning of tuning in to the body, allowing the body to speak. The needles aid the concentration and awareness, but once that is achieved, maybe they are no longer necessary.

One of the classical medical texts describes the action of the needles in an acupuncture treatment as 'attracting the spirit'. This can also be described as attracting the mind or consciousness. In masssage, movement or simply by thought, if we can focus our consciousness we can begin our own healing. We can learn to develop awareness in our bodies, taking the time and space to relax and release, to listen and look within, reclaiming the wisdom of the body, which we all have, but are usually too busy to notice.

The aim of this book is to give an introduction to the ideas behind Chinese medicine and some simple ways to put them into practice. These ideas are the same whether applied to acupuncture, herbal medicine, massage, diet or exercise. They are the same whether practised in China, Japan, Vietnam or any other country. There have been countless schools and traditions, some of which have claimed to be the only true way, but at its root it is the same medicine.

Developed long before its written history, the first Chinese medical texts date from the 3rd century BCE. Many of the Daoist and Confucian ideas that inform the early medical texts date from the 6th century BCE. From that time, Chinese medicine has spread throughout much of the Far East, and was introduced into Japan by Buddhist scholars in the 8th century CE. Many Japanese schools would claim that it is they who have kept to its true ancient form. During the 17th century acupuncture became an accepted occupation for the blind in Japan, the practitioners inevitably obtaining a highly developed sense of touch. The Japanese tradition has generally stressed subtle energetics, choosing finer needles and a more delicate approach.

Traditional medicine went into decline in both China and Japan with the introduction of Western scientific medicine, but has regained some popularity in recent decades. Postrevolution China encouraged traditional medicine and Western medicine to develop hand in hand, though creating a rift between the practice of traditional medicine and its Daoist and Confucian roots, which were frowned upon by the state. Official textbooks imported to the West tended to reflect the party line.

In the 17th century Jesuit missionaries in China and Dutch traders to Japan brought back reports of this exotic form of medicine, but it was not until the publication of Soulie de Morant's *L'Acupuncture chinoise* (1939–41) that acupuncture was studied seriously in the West. Its infiltration into the rest of Europe tended to be among those individuals already involved in the fringes of medicine – osteopaths, naturopaths and homeopaths – who found that this system, though foreign in its language, expressed similar concepts to their own.

After President Nixon's historic visit to China in the early 1970s, and with China opening its doors to the West, many sensationalist reports of acupuncture anaesthesia and pain control hit the headlines. This inspired much research and speculation, but focused attention solely on acupuncture and its ability to relieve pain. The wider implications of Chinese medicine still awaited discovery.

In the past 25 years acupuncture, herbal medicine, macrobiotics, shiatsu massage, tai ji quan, qi gong and many other Far Eastern traditional health care practices have become accepted in the West. More and more people are beginning to work with diet, exercise and many other do-it-yourself therapies to aid their own self-healing. But for many, Chinese medicine has remained in the domain of the expert, its language and cultural basis making it appear remote and inaccessible. But Chinese medicine can offer simple techniques to balance our energy and to motivate our inner healing potential. It is a tradition full of practical everyday wisdom, much of which has been hidden by its apparent obscurity and unfamiliarity.

Exercise, breathing techniques, massage and diet have traditionally formed an important part of mainstream medicine in China and are incorporated into the lives of millions of people in the East. When I attended the public baths in Japan, the women massaged each other's backs and shoulders while catching up on the day's gossip. It was an integral part of their daily lives. In China millions exercise daily in the parks and squares, each performing their individual practice.

Chinese medicine is unique in being an ancient healing system, based on shamanism and earth magic, that has survived intact into the modern scientific era, where it has been held up to rigorous clinical trials both in China and in the West. An understanding of this tradition can help us to respect the intelligence in nature and to reclaim the wisdom of the body, not to return to a more primitive system but to include our natural body-knowing in the medicine of the future. We can embrace the advances of modern science without losing our common sense. The ancient systems of healing that are currently re-emerging can help to remind us of those simple truths we once knew; guiding us back to a more natural use of energy, on a bodily and by extension planetary level. It is my hope that this book will help to make the insights of this wonderful system more accessible.

In Part 1 we will look at the philosophy behind the medicine, based in the Daoism and Confucianism which both influenced the early medical texts. These ideas embrace the theory of yin yang and the five elements and show how these principles underlie the functions of the internal organs. Though dating from 2nd century BCE, the descriptions of the anatomical organs are remarkably close to those of a much later scientific medicine, but they should not been seen as identical in function. When talking of the heart, the early medical texts may be referring to the mind or the intelligence;

in modern Japanese, the two terms are still interchangeable. The heart can be used to define the emotions in the West, but in the West we do not expect to come across this terminology in a medical text! To treat a heart condition in Chinese medicine, one is equally as likely to concentrate on the emotional state as on the physical. Sometimes there is very little distinction made; one being seen as a continuum of the other.

Chinese medical terminology is symbolic, and attempts in modern China to make the medicine accessible to the Western scientific mind have often complicated matters by neglecting to draw attention to this. The spleen in Chinese medicine is not just the obscure little organ that most of us are hard-pressed to define – either its position or its function – but the centre of all digestion and transformation of food to energy, the absorption and digestion of ideas, as well as a prime player in the production of blood. In Part 1 we will attempt to illustrate these functions, and see how the interactions of the five elements form a basis for this symbolism. The order in which the elements are presented may change according to the context. There is no fixed pattern, just a continual interplay.

In Part 2 we will look at the bodily landscape, with a brief introduction to the meridian system, and a closer look at some of the primary meridians and points. The names of acupuncture points are given where they help us to under-stand the function. Translations from the Chinese are often difficult, and where no English translation is adequate, I have used the Chinese term. Chinese characters often include a variety of possible interpretations and it is the interplay of these different meanings that gives a richness to the concepts.

This meridian system of subtle energy pathways forms the basis for acupuncture, shiatsu, massage, exercise and even herbal medicine. A basic understanding of the pathways can make a vast difference to the practice of many Eastern disciplines, rendering the obscure and impenetrable accessible and straightforward. A simple qi gong movement becomes full of purpose when you know why you are doing it; the massage of an acupuncture point becomes more potent when you understand the function of the meridian of which it is a part. I have tried to keep this section simple – but there is much new information. It may be most useful when used as reference for Parts 3–5.

Parts 3–5 introduce simple self-help techniques. Part 3 suggests exercises and breathing techniques for general health and balance. Part 4 addresses each of five elements and their related internal organs and meridians, suggesting massage, exercise and meditation techniques and looking at emotional tendencies. Part 5 looks at some common problems and begins to differentiate them in terms of Chinese medicine, suggesting treatments and offering simple advice.

GLOSSARY

chong mai	the penetrating vessel – the third of the eight extraordinary meridians; creating a surge of life through the conjunction of yin and yang
dai mai	the girdle vessel – the fourth of the eight extraordinary meridians; the horizontal belt, creating volume and space
dan tian	cinnabar field, or field of elixir; the three energy centres located at the lower abdomen, the heart and the brow
Dao	the way – to follow the Dao, to live according to your true nature
du mai	the governor vessel – first of the eight extraordinary meridians; the primary yang meridian
hun	the spiritual aspect related to the liver and the wood element – the individual soul, manifesting in dreams, imagination, creativity
ming men	the gate of life – the alchemical fire of the lower dan tian, the beginning of all transformation and transmutation; the acupuncture point ming men, du mai 4, is on the spine at the level of the waist (between lumber vertebrae 2 and 3)

moxa/moxibustion	the burning of a herb (artemisia vulgaris) to warm and strengthen a particular acupuncture point or area of weakness
po	the spiritual aspect related to the lungs and metal – the intelligence of the body
qi gong	working with qi – movement and visualisation to stimulate the subtle energy channels and centres
qiao mai	yin and yang qiao mai – two of the eight extraordinary meridians which govern the rhythms and cycles of yin and yang
ren mai	the conception vessel – the primary yin meridian; the second of the eight extraordinary meridians
tai ji quan	(tai chi chuan) a series of movements to balance the meridian system and strengthen the body
wei mai	yin and yang wei mai, two of the eight extraordinary meridians; the yin wei preserves the yin and blood, the yang wei organises the yang and the qi
yi	the spiritual aspect of the spleen and the earth element – purpose, the way in which we receive external ideas and influences

PART 1

THE PHILOSOPHY
OF CHINESE MEDICINE

Understanding the Body

HEAVEN AND EARTH

Chinese medicine sees all life as an interplay of the energies of heaven and earth. If these energies are in balance, there is health, if they are out of balance there is illness. This is not a static balance of opposing forces cancelling each other out but a dynamic interaction, constantly able to adapt and change to each new circumstance.

Earth brings form and matter, condensation and density. It is our source of nourishment. In Chinese medicine it is known as yin. The earth not only provides nourishment through the food that we eat but also through the energies that are drawn up through our feet to nourish and cool the body via the yin meridians.

Heaven brings heat, light and expansion, and is known as yang. The energy of heaven and of the sun flow downwards in the yang meridians, creating movement and warmth, just as a plant draws water and food from the earth and energy for its transformations from the sun.

The interplay of yin and yang is at the heart of all ancient Chinese thought, and the idea of constant change and mutual dependency of opposing forces is at the heart of the medicine. Yin and yang serve as a symbolic reminder of the need for balance. The yin yang symbol suggests self-regulation, homeostasis, the body as a self-regulating system in a perpetual state of flux. In Chinese medicine change and adaptation are seen as the most important factors determining physical, emotional and spiritual health.

The four seasons are a constant reminder from nature of the inevitability of change: of growth, flowering, harvesting, decline and decay, allowing rebirth and a continuity of the cycle. The system of the five elements, or more correctly the five expressions of movement, on which the early medicine is based, comes from a close observation of these changes in energy throughout the natural yearly cycles of growth and decline, change and transformation.

Our bodies are part of the earth, our spirit part of heaven, and it is the observation of the interaction of yin and yang, heaven and earth, and the energetic fluctuation of the five elements within ourselves that can help us regain our body-knowing.

YIN YANG AND THE FOUR SEASONS

Heaven and earth, yin and yang interact to create the four seasons. Yang, representing heat, light, sun, outward movement and manifestation is characterised by the spring and summer, the time of heat and light and growth. Yin, representing darkness, cold, inward movement and potential, is characterised by the autumn and winter, the time for decline and preservation.

Spring is the time of young yang, full of vitality, energy and life; summer of old yang, of maturity, flourishing, bearing fruit. Spring and summer are the seasons when energy is moving upwards and outwards, expanding with heat and light. In the autumn there is a closing in, a darkening of the light, a time of harvesting and preparing for withdrawal. In winter the energy is hidden within, like a seed hidden within the earth, a time of hibernation, conservation, storage.

These four movements, outwards and upwards, inwards and downwards are stabilised by a fifth, a central, pivotal force which balances the others. These five movements, usually translated as the five elements, or the five phases, form the basis of the complex system of resonances or correspondences that are at the core of Oriental medicine.

The expanding energy of spring, with its ability to burst

outer

movement

space

expansion

heat

energy

spirit

heaven

yang

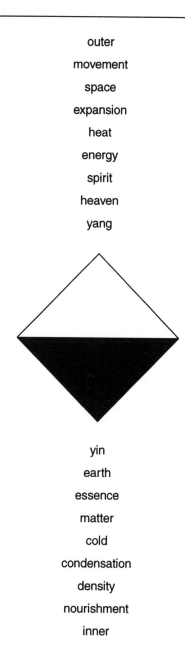

yin

earth

essence

matter

cold

condensation

density

nourishment

inner

Table 1: Yin and Yang

through restrictions and reach up towards the light, is called wood. Not the wood of a solid, static lump of timber, but the ability of a seed to penetrate the earth and grow towards the light, the pliable yielding strength of the willow, able to bend with the wind and not break. Its colour is the vibrant green of living plants.

Its opposite is the heavy contracting energy of autumn, the ability to concentrate and condense, to conserve and preserve. It is seen in nature as the energy of metal, symbolising all that is contracted, condensed and made precious within the earth. It is the return to the earth, and its colour is white, the colour of death and of ghosts.

In summer energy moves upwards towards heaven. The sun is closest to the earth, and it is symbolised by the element fire. From ancient times fires were used in ritual to show man's relation to the gods, and fire represents the spirit, the aspiration towards the other, the release of energy from matter. Its colour is red, the colour, in China, of heaven.

In winter energy descends into the depths. Animals hibernate to conserve energy and food resources. Its movement is symbolised by water, cold, dark, always finding the lowest point. Its colour is the blue/black of the abyss.

The central pivot is the energy of earth, constantly rotating on its axis and holding the other forces in balance. Its colour is the yellow of harvested grains. Its function is that of change and transformation, and it is seen as the change of season, and particularly the time of late summer, of harvest, when there is a major change of energy from the expansion of yang in the summer to the withdrawal towards yin.

Fire and water balance each other on the vertical or heavenly axis, the downward, cooling energy of water constantly controlling the tendency of fire to flare up and burn out; the warmth of fire bringing life and movement to water with its tendency to freeze up and stagnate. Fire and water are the primal manifestations of yin and yang on the earth, and their constant interaction creates life. No life can exist without fire and water, and it is the particular balance of fire and water on our planet that makes human life possible.

Wood and metal form the horizontal or earthly axis. Both

represent properties of life on earth, one generation and birth, the other decline and decay. And both are essential for life. There can be no spring without autumn and winter, no germination without a seed falling to the earth. No expansion unless there has first been a contraction. The contrasting movements of wood and metal allow a continual flow of energy between fire and water, creating a natural cycle where there had been only a pull of opposites.

The Chinese considered the seasonal changes to be the most instructive teacher on how to change and flow with the circumstances of life: not to want summer when it is autumn, or spring before winter has made its necessary preparations. The cycle of the year teaches us the inevitability of change and an acceptance of the equality of all things. We may prefer spring to winter, but observation of the seasons teaches us that we cannot have one without the other. The harder the winter the more beautiful the spring.

The Japanese developed a culture around the love of simplicity, the beauty of melancholy, a quiet, dignified acceptance of what is. Autumn is often the time of year that the Japanese prefer, explaining that it most closely expresses their national soul. But maybe it is not always balanced with an appreciation of the expansion of life, of individuality, of creativity, and occasionally these underdeveloped aspects erupt in violence and passion. The West, on the other hand, tends to have favoured growth and expansion on all levels, neglecting the necessary balance of simplicity and stillness; our body/minds becoming increasingly burnt up, stressed out until we are finally unable to rest, sleep, restore, rejuvenate.

In our bodies and in our lives we need to balance the yin and yang, not by creating a false state of equilibrium and inertia, but by constantly adapting and changing to the circumstances of life. When it is time to be active we are active, when it is time to rest, we rest; balancing expansion with contraction, movement with stillness and allowing life to flow through us without resistance.

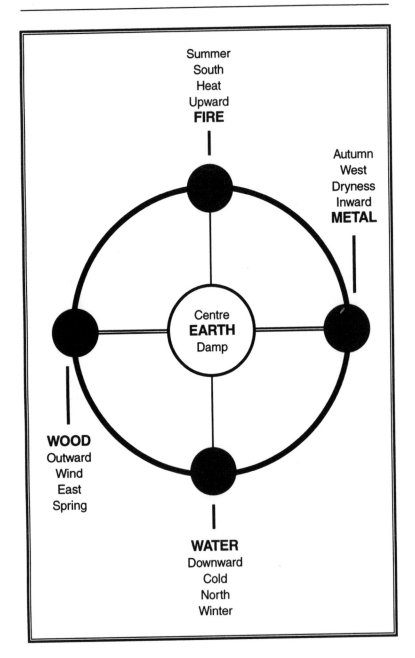

Table 2: The Five Elements

THE FIVE ELEMENTS

WOOD

The wood phase is related to the expansive energy of spring, its direction is east, the direction of the rising sun. It is associated with the wind, which brings motion and change. In the body it is the muscles and tendons giving movement and pliability; the eyes giving clear sight; the organs and channels of the liver and gall-bladder allowing freeflow of blood and energy. In health it is uninterrupted change and flow, ability to adapt, physically and emotionally to external circumstances. In illness, it may be excessive movement, tremors and shaking, fits and convulsions, or conversely, blockage, stuckness, inability to move forward in life. Emotionally, the violent upward, outward movement of wood energy is expressed as anger. Lack of this element can cause the inner blockage of frustration, repression and certain types of depression.

FIRE

The fire element is related to midsummer, its direction is south and its associated climate is heat. Within the body, it controls the heart, the blood and the cardiovascular system, though most ancient texts stress the importance of the heart and the fire element as the home of the spirits. When the fire element is balanced, there is peace and harmony in the body; when it is unbalanced there is agitation, insomnia, palpitations. The emotion corresponding to the heart and to fire is joy, a quiet, inner, peaceful joy. In imbalance it is over-excitement, excess joy, a constant need for stimulation and excitement, leading in the extreme to mania.

Fire and wood are the two yang elements, and the heart and the liver energies both have a tendency to flare up out of control. Most of their pathologies are those of excess rather than deficiency. As their energies move upwards and outwards, symptoms often occur at the top of the body, with for example, headaches, eye problems or too much thinking.

METAL

The condensing, contracting energy of metal and the autumn season is related to dryness and the west, the direction of the setting sun. In the body it is responsible for extracting that which is of value, and eliminating that which is not. Its organs and channels are the lung and large intestine; its body parts are the skin and body hair, or pores. Emotionally, this inward, condensing movement is grief and sadness, causing constriction and sinking particularly of the lungs and the chest. It may be because Chinese medicine recognises this relationship between the lungs and the skin, as seen so often in cases of asthma and eczema, and between lung problems and grief and sadness, that it is so successful in treating these conditions. Clinically, many cases of eczema, psoriasis and other skin problems are seen to be related to the lung and colon, often first occurring along these channels. Problems in the metal element are often related to holding on, not letting go, not responding to the need to withdraw and to conserve.

WATER

The water element is related to winter and to midnight, to darkness and withdrawal. Its climate is cold and its direction the north. In the body, water cools and descends, constantly balancing the heating upward movement of fire; it controls all that is innermost, hidden and secret. In the organs and channels it is the kidneys and bladder, controlling water distribution, reabsorption and elimination. But to the Chinese the kidneys have a more far-reaching function. Being a double organ, the kidneys are seen as the primal balance of yin and yang within the body. They control all the energy in the lower abdomen, and are responsible for reproduction and growth. Kidney yin and kidney yang, or kidney fire and kidney water, must be kept in balance both to prolong life and to create new life. Chinese alchemy uses these symbols of fire and water in the depths of the body as a basis for transformation and transmutation of energies and substances.

The emotion linked with water is fear.

EARTH

The earth is the centre, nourishing and balancing the other elements. Its climate is humidity and dampness, its season the time of harvest, or the change of one season into another. Its movement is rotation. In the body it is the spleen and stomach; that which accepts, transforms and transports nourishment. It governs the flesh and the shape of the body. A deficiency of the spleen and stomach means that we do not transform and absorb food efficiently. Either we are unable to transform food into flesh, with a tendency to lose weight, or we are unable to transform food into energy, so that we store and put on weight, but do not transform and release. Unless there are obvious eating disorders, weight problems do not tend to be treated by diet in Chinese medicine, but rather by helping the body's ability to absorb and transform. If the body is large, slow and sluggish, it will need to be moved and warmed; if the body is thin and wiry it needs to be calmed down and encouraged to rest and relax.

In the emotions the earth element governs the ability for reflective thought, to turn things around in the mind. Pathologically this can become worry and obsession.

THE FIVE INTERNAL ORGANS

The physiology of the five internal organs is based on the resonances of the five elements, and forms the basis of Chinese medicine, whether acupuncture, herbs, diet or exercise. The five solid organs of the heart, the kidneys, the spleen, the lungs and the liver carry out the essential roles of production, transformation and regulation of blood and qi (energy), the function of each organ spreading throughout the body via a subtle network of channels. They are mutually dependent, generating and controlling.

Taking the most common phrases from the Chinese medical classics to describe the functions of these five organs, we can slowly build a picture of the whole body.

THE HEART

'The heart is the emperor and ruler'

Although the Chinese system is essentially one of mutual dependency, the heart still retains this prime position as the emperor. Though later texts may have stressed the anatomical importance of the heart as an organ, the central pump bringing life to all parts of the body, the more ancient texts such as the *Nei Jing*, 'The Yellow Emperor's Classic of Internal Medicine', and the *Dao de Jing*, 'The Way and its Power', stress the heart as the spiritual and emotional centre of the body, bringing the understanding that if the heart is at rest, the body can function well; if the heart is agitated, the body cannot function well.

In the stress and anxiety of the modern world, these ancient words have a potent message and they refer to more than the physical heart. The heart in its role as emperor occupies the 'central palace', the point in the centre of the chest associated with the heart chakra. This centre is the void, the empty space within that allows the body to be at rest, allows the rhythms of the heart and lungs to regulate and circulate the blood and energy throughout the body.

'The heart stores the spirits'

If the heart is at rest, the spirits can be stored. If the heart is not empty but full of agitation, the spirits cannot settle and there will be restlessness, insomnia, palpitations. Spirit is seen in the shine of the eye, the glow of the face and, whatever the presenting symptoms, there is obviously more chance of a successful cure if the spirit is good. An excess of spirit can be seen in cases of hyperactivity and mania. In this way the spirit may be seen as a kind of intelligence and a clarity of mind. Modern texts equate the spirit with the mind and consciousness, whereas the ancient texts suggest a multitude of spirits which pour down their influence from heaven. We only have to be still enough and open enough to receive them. Meditation calms the heart and stills the mind and allows this heavenly influx of spirits.

'The heart governs the blood and the vessels'

The heart distributes nutrition and energy to all the cells of the body via the network of blood vessels. Each of the five organs has its own function in maintaining the quality and quantity of blood, but the heart moves it and gives it vitality and spirit. The classical texts suggest that the red colour of blood is the imprint of the fire of the heart – the mark of the spirit. If the blood is insufficient in either quantity or quality this may also affect the mind or the spirit, and many cases of restlessness and insomnia may be due to some kind of blood deficiency.

'The heart governs speech'

When the five emotions are in balance and the mind is clear, so the speech will be clear. A disturbed heart manifests in loud speech, shouting, excessive laughing or giggling. The heart channel attaches to the root of the tongue, affecting its movement. And shock, which blocks the energy of the heart and its channel, may cause an inability to speak; a paralysis of the tongue which may be temporary or in rare cases permanent.

An enlarged, protruding tongue that is difficult to move is often associated with blockage in the heart and its channels; in these cases the heart is said to be misted or clouded, bringing a lack of clarity to the mind and dullness to the spirit. The speech will be slurred and slow. These kinds of effects can be seen in the use of various mood-altering drugs, which all ultimately damage the heart and the spirit.

'The heart is averse to heat'

Heat can over-excite and over-stimulate the heart and its channels; the source of the heat may be internal, from within the body, or external. Heat within the body can be caused by an unbalanced diet, particularly too much alcohol, spicy or fried foods, but also from emotional causes, particularly an excess of anger. Heat within the body may be expressed as uncontrolled anger or rage, whereas long-standing repression of anger will eventually create heat and will damage the heart and the spirit.

Many of the emotional disturbances of menopause are caused by a false heat generated when the cooling yin qualities and the energising yang qualities in the body are struggling to create a new order within a changed environment. Typical mood swings occur as the fire and water energies in the body attempt to restore equilibrium.

'The heart and kidneys are mutually dependent'

We have already seen the importance of the balance between the fire and water energies, and in the body many pathologies come from an imbalance between the heart and the kidneys. The water must be strong enough to control the tendency of fire energy to blaze upwards. The kidneys are the root and have a grounding, stabilising effect, but without the warmth of fire the water would have no life, no ability to transform. This constant interplay between heart and kidneys, fire and water, spirit and essence forms the basis of the innermost workings of life, and they are joined in the term shao yin, or lesser yin, describing that which is most internal, most deep and most precious. As a shao yin couple, the kidneys represent that which governs the innermost structure of life while the heart governs the expansion of that energy, outwards and upwards into manifestation, just as the winter is the time for the development of inner structure and the summer the time for outward manifestation. We will see more of this balance as we go on to look more deeply at the functions of the kidneys.

'The heart is connected with the small intestine'

Each of the five inner organs (heart, kidneys, liver, lungs, spleen) is connected with a coupled organ in a yin/yang or interior/exterior relationship. The heart is connected with the small intestine and they are both governed by the fire element. It is the fire of the small intestine that facilitates the separation of food received from the stomach into its pure (to be assimilated) and impure (to be evacuated) aspects. Fire gives this ability to distinguish what is useful from what is not – and some would say that the small intestine is able to separate what is useful from what is not useful on the physical level while the heart does so on the emotional level.

THE KIDNEYS

'The kidneys store essence'

The spirit of the heart must be grounded by the essence of the kidneys. This essence, or jing, is the most refined substance of our material body, governing all aspects of reproduction, growth and development. It forms the basis of our constitutional energy and it is said that we all inherit a certain amount of jing essence from our parents; when this supply is exhausted we die. Kidney essence is considered irreplaceable in the medical texts – it can be conserved but not made, though alchemists throughout the centuries have claimed that their various methods, whether external, with pills and potions, or internal, with breathing and meditation techniques, have increased the quality and quantity of kidney essence.

The medical tradition tends to prefer conservation and advises against loss of essence, particularly through excess sex for men and too many childbirths for women. Sperm is the most obvious physical counterpart of pure essence, and loss of sperm is seen as a loss of jing, hence the stress on control of ejaculation in intercourse, both to preserve the essence of the male and to free the woman from unwanted pregnancy. These practices may be taken further into a kind of sexual alchemy where the blending of male and female essences during intercourse become enriching rather than depleting and there is a perfect balance of the essence of the kidneys and the spirit of the heart.

'Essence generates qi, qi generates spirit'

Essence (jing), energy (qi) and spirit (shen), are known as the Three Treasures and form the basis of every energetic transformation in the body. Essence gives the material basis, qi the energetic movement, spirit the intelligence. We separate them in order to attempt to understand them, but they are in fact inseparable; jing cannot exist without shen, it would be inert matter; shen could not exist without jing, it would be pure spirit and unable to stay in the body. It is this combination of jing and shen, essence and spirit, that gives life. In conception it is the essence of the father combining with the essence of the mother that gives a new form, but it is not until this form is combined with spirit that there is life.

Essence is the liquid, material matrix which provides the raw ingredients of life; spirit is the heavenly spark which organises and gives intelligence; qi is the mechanism that makes this possible. It is the breath, the vitality, that which joins fire and water, yin and yang, heaven and earth. It moves, warms, protects and transforms.

The conservation and refining of essence is of vital importance for the generation of qi; the purification and harmonising of qi is vital for the radiance of the spirit. These are natural processes which take place in the body all the time, though many Chinese meditation practices aim to aid this process of mutual generation, making it more efficient. But as always, care must be taken to keep a balance. Certain spiritual practices over-emphasise spirit to the detriment of matter, but while in the physical body it is necessary that the Three Treasures work together in balance and harmony.

'The kidneys rule water'

Water dampens, fertilises and penetrates to the depths, and its function in the body is the same as its function in nature. The kidneys therefore govern moisture, fertility and the ability to have roots. They keep liquids in the right proportion and in the right place, retaining and drawing downwards. The kidneys must ensure that there is no leakage of water or precious fluids and they are responsible for sealing and closing against loss of essence, whether through excess urination, sweating, crying or a running nose. They work with all the other organs in controlling liquids throughout the body.

'The kidneys govern the bones and marrow'

The kidneys are the base, the root and the deep structure of the body. The yang aspect is represented by the bones, giving stability, solidity, structure; the yin aspect by the marrow, with its richness and fluidity within the bones. From this association with the bones and marrow comes the important connection between the kidneys, the spinal cord and the brain. The brain is called the 'sea of marrow' and it is the quality of marrow in the brain, the combination of essence and spirit, that gives clarity of thought and wisdom.

Externally the bones manifest as the teeth, and the state of the teeth is a good measure of the state of the kidneys; the marrow manifests in the condition of the hair. As the kidney essence becomes diminished in old age the teeth and hair decline.

'The kidneys control the fire of the gate of life'

The gate of life or the gate of destiny, ming men, is the place of 'original qi' and the yang of the kidneys, our connection with the root of our life and our true nature. The fire of the gate of life allows all energetic transformations, and figures centrally in inner alchemical practices. It is often depicted as a cauldron in which the liquid and essence of kidney yin is heated by the fire of kidney yang.

At the centre of the back, between the kidneys, there is an acupuncture point called ming men, the gate of life. It is commonly used in acupuncture, massage and exercise to strengthen the kidneys, promote energy production and to warm and invigorate the whole body. Cold and weakness in this area suggests a deficency in the yang of the kidneys.

'The kidneys are the root of former heaven'

'The root of former heaven' is a poetic description of that which comes with us at birth. It is the energetic tendencies that we inherit both from the combination of the essences of our parents and from our own individual intrinsic nature. It is more easily understood when compared with 'the root of later heaven' which refers to the energy generated by the spleen and stomach and is a combination of the food that we eat and the air that we breathe. Former heaven is what we come with, later heaven is what we make of it. This brings us back to the notion that we cannot do much to change our inherited constitution, but we can do everything to control the food that we eat and the way that we breathe – thus making sure that we get the most out of what we have got. If our inherited energy is not strong, we must take more care with diet and exercise.

'The kidneys govern reproduction'

The first chapter of the *Nei Jing Su Wen*, the first part of *The Yellow Emperor's Classic of Internal Medicine*, describes the cycles of fertility in men and women, and these cycles correspond to the maturing and declining of the kidney energy. In women the cycles are of seven years, the first marking the growth of the hair and the renewal of the teeth, both, as we have seen, an external manifestation of the power of the kidneys; at 14 there is the beginning of menstruation and the onset of fertility; at 21 the wisdom teeth grow and the woman becomes mature. At 28, the bones are solid, the hair reaches its full length, the body is strong and powerful. At 35 the energy begins to decline, at 42 the yin essence no longer reaches the top of the body, the face begins to wrinkle and the strength of the hair declines. At 49 fertility is exhausted and she can no longer have children.

The cycles in the male follow eight years, with the first cycle bringing the growth of hair and the renewal of teeth as with the woman. The second cycle at 16 brings fertility, with the rise of the qi of the kidneys allowing emission of sperm (jing). At 24 the bones are powerful and the wisdom teeth grow, at 32 there is full strength and vigour. Decline begins at 40 when the qi of the kidneys grows weaker, the hair begins to fall out and the teeth 'dry out'. At 48 the essence no longer reaches the top of the body and the hair begins to whiten, the face becomes wrinkled and dry. At 56 there is the first mention of the liver energy which in the male combines with the qi of the kidneys to sustain erection. At this time it begins to decline, making all movement more difficult. At 64, fertility is exhausted, the sperm (jing) is less, the teeth and hair fall out.

This graphic description of the rise and fall of vitality written over 2,000 years ago is particularly interesting in its portrayal of the kidneys as the key to fertility and reproduction. Although other organs play their part, particularly the liver, if the kidneys' energy is not strong there will be problems with reproduction. Most cases of infertility and impotence are treated via the kidneys.

'The kidneys are connected with the bladder'

Both governed by the element water, the kidneys and bladder form an internal/external partnership in the transformation, reabsorption and excretion of water. The bladder meridian is called the great yang or tai yang, its pathway extending from the eyes, penetrating the brain, and following a double pathway down the back, with two channels either side of the spine. It is on the bladder meridian that all the internal organs have their main treatment points, which relate closely to the nervous connections of the organs with the spinal cord. It is interesting that the Chinese were aware of these connections some 300 years BCE. Misalignment of vertebrae or tension in the muscles either side of the spine can cause problems with the related internal organs.

THE SPLEEN

'The spleen governs the centre, earth'

The vertical axis of the heart and the kidneys is mediated by the central movement of the earth. The properties of the earth are to take in and give out, to take in seeds and to give out a harvest, and within the body the spleen is the central place where food is received, transformed and redistributed. The spleen earth in the body is the 'central pivot', revolving like a central turn-table, to receive and distribute. The spleen and stomach, almost inseparable as a couple in Chinese medicine, are often called the messenger· and the marketplace, the storehouses and granaries, taking in and giving out food and nourishment.

The energies of the stomach and spleen also govern those aspects of the psyche concerned with the ability to take in, transform and move on, to be all-encompassing, adaptable, able to change with the seasons of life.

'The spleen governs movement and transformation'

The stomach takes in the raw ingredients of nutrition; the spleen must transform those raw ingredients into a usable energy and distribute it amongst the other organs. From its central place the spleen provides nourishment on a gross and subtle level, refining the most subtle energies from food and raising them to the level of the heart and lungs, the head and the brain to feed the sense organs and the psyche; the less subtle are distributed to the other organs, to the flesh and the muscles.

'The spleen governs the muscles and flesh'

The liver controls the flexibility of the muscles, but the spleen governs their shape and size, in much the same way as it controls the shape and size of the whole body. All problems with the shape and size of the body, whether excess or deficiency, are problems of the spleen and stomach. It is the body's ability to act as the earth – to receive, to transform and to nourish – that tends to go wrong and to create various problems with the muscles and flesh. Some people take in well but are unable to absorb. Others take in, transform to flesh, but not to energy. Yet others refuse to take in at all, unable to receive, some can never receive enough.

But in all this it is vital to remember that the needs of each individual are different, depending on their body type and their underlying energetic tendencies, and therefore any sweeping generalisations about diet and weight are likely to be useless. In diet it is vital to know yourself, to know your type and to understand what works for you.

'The spleen manages blood'

All the organs have a particular role in the creation and maintenance of blood. The spleen is responsible for managing or controlling blood, both for distributing nutrition and for keeping blood in its proper place. Deficiency in blood quality, for example types of anaemia, may be a deficiency in the spleen's ability to transform and absorb nutrients. If the diet is balanced and sufficient, the use of supplements may not always be helpful, as the body's inability to absorb may be at the root of the problem. The spleen's central position also makes it responsible for holding things in their proper place, thus all haemorrhages or seepage of blood are seen as a deficiency of spleen energy.

'Spleen qi governs upbearing'

The central rotation of the earth energy creates a subtle gravitational pull which keeps the organs in their place. All forms of prolapse are therefore said to be caused by a deficiency of the energy of the spleen.

'The spleen is the root of later heaven'

As the kidneys are the root of pre-heaven, governing all that is inherited at birth, the spleen is the root of later heaven, and governs the energetic transformation that takes place on the more mundane, day-to-day level: the intake of food, the transformation of food to energy, the intake of air, and the uptake of oxygen by the blood. It is the combination of energy and essence from food with the energy from the air we breathe that gives the nutritional energy that circulates in the acupuncture meridians and maintains the body.

The body's innate ability to carry out these transformations may be constitutional and therefore controlled by pre-heavenly energy and the kidneys. As it is thought that little can be done to change these constitutional tendencies, many schools of medicine have developed which treat only the stomach and spleen – assuming that if these organs are functioning well, everything else will follow.

'Spleen qi flows to the mouth'

Each organ has its appropriate orifice, and the one that most obviously relates to the spleen is the mouth. Its sense is therefore the sense of taste. Each organ also has its own particular taste, the liver acid, the heart bitter, the lung pungent, the kidney salty and the spleen sweet. These five tastes must be balanced in the diet, and they play a vital part in all Far Eastern methods of dietary and herbal medicine.

The five tastes are said to be balanced in the spleen, which differentiates and distributes the subtle taste of foods to the appropriate organ. Therefore the acid taste enhances the attributes of the liver, but the liver may be damaged by an excess of acid; the kidneys are invigorated by the salty taste, but too much salt can harm the kidneys. Coffee is an example of the bitter taste that stimulates the heart, but which can easily over-stimulate in excess, causing palpitations or insomnia.

Both Chinese and Japanese cuisines are based on a balance of the five tastes within each meal. A balance of colour is also important, as the colour of food also shows its energetic attributes.

'The spleen is averse to dampness'

All the organs are affected by an excess of their related climate, and the spleen is injured by dampness. As the climate appropriate to the earth element, it is essential for all fertility and growth, but an excess of dampness causes the earth to be waterlogged. The ability to move and transform, those vital yang qualities of the spleen, are damaged. Dampness in the spleen will cause an inability to transform fluids, creating a build-up of fluids in the body leading to oedema, or the creation of mucus and phlegm. The presence of phlegm in the body slows down the transformation processes even more, and the body becomes heavy and sluggish.

'The spleen is connected with the stomach'

We have seen that the spleen is closely related to its earth element partner, the stomach. These two organs work together in all aspects of digestion and assimilation, the spleen dealing with the more energetic aspects of food, the stomach with the more physical. The spleen distributes the fine energies from food to the five internal organs, the stomach sends the more physical food into the gut for further assimilation and finally excretion. The stomach meridian is the only yang meridian to flow down the front of the body. Although the stomach is considered to be a yang organ, it is also involved with nutrition, and the fact that its meridian flows in this more yin area of the body, actually passing through the nipples, shows another facet to the stomach's role in providing nourishment. It is the stomach meridian that is generally treated in lactation difficulties.

THE LIVER

'The liver governs freeflow'

The energy of the liver spreads out and rises upwards. It allows free circulation and diffusion of qi and blood throughout the whole body. It is differentiated from the circulating ability of the heart and the regulation of that circulation by the lungs, in that its movement is dynamic; based in the water of the kidneys the liver wood rises upwards and outwards expressing the vitality and growth of the life force in the spring.

Liver problems tend to manifest as an excess of upward and outward movement, with headaches, agitation and irritability, or in a lack of that movement, with blockage, stuckness and depression. The characteristic of this kind of stuckness is that the force of the liver may suddenly break through in an uprush of energy, manifesting as anger or migraine-type headaches. Typical liver symptoms are violent; they come and go, move around and are difficult to pin down.

They are like the wind, moving, changing, creating chaos or bringing the lifegiving quality of movement and change to that which is stuck and in decline.

This energetic freeflow is vital in terms of emotional balance. In the Chinese classics the emotions are often compared to the wind. They must be allowed to flow freely, like the wind through a flute. Only when they are stopped, blocked or over-indulged do they create problems. Learning to observe the emotions with detachment, allowing them to come and go without too much identification with them is an important step in healthy energetic balance. The emotions are nothing other than a movement of energy. If emotions are blocked, there is a stoppage in the energy associated with them, which can in turn create physical problems.

Anger, the emotion associated with the liver, is an upward, outward movement of qi. In excess, anger can dissipate energy, creating heat and fire, and damaging the yin and the fluids. If blocked, anger will cause the energy to be knotted and stuck, creating pains in the ribs and sides, and a lack of freeflow in the abdomen, causing, for example, digestive and menstrual problems.

This concept of freeflow is central to all liver functions, and a lack of freeflow is at the root of liver pathologies.

'The liver stores the blood'

Movement and freeflow are the yang aspects of the liver; the yin aspect is the ability to store blood. But storing is an active process, keeping the quality and the quantity of the blood intact. This combination of the functions of freeflow and blood storage makes the liver of primary importance in treating menstrual disorders, particularly premenstrual symptoms, with headache and irritability, and stuckness and blockage in the menstrual flow causing pain.

The Chinese medical classics say that when the body is at rest, the blood returns to the liver: sleep and dreams are therefore also related to this function of the liver, which we will see in more detail when we look at the spirits of the organs. Blood or yin are needed to ground the yang energy and the spirits. If the blood is deficient, either in quality or quantity, the yang will rise, possibly causing headaches and dizziness, agitation and restless sleep.

The liver is responsible for blood supply to the muscles, its related body part, and to the eyes, its related orifice. Therefore cramps and spasms in the muscles, dry, itchy eyes or blurred vision are often seen as a deficiency of the blood of the liver. Stiffness in the joints and any other problems to do with the general movement of the body may also be a sign of liver blood deficiency.

'The liver governs physical movement'

In governing muscles and tendons, the liver by extension controls all physical movement: bending and stretching, walking and running, but also the small articulations that allow for precision. As we have seen, it is the liver's function of freeflow and its ability to store blood that allow the muscles to be nourished, and it is by nourishment that the muscles are able to function.

It is important to remember that the liver represents the wood element in the body, and the climate of wind. Many liver symptoms can be compared to the action of the wind and the properties of the wood element in nature. If there is insufficient blood in the liver there may be trembling and shaking in the limbs, or the body may become stiff and unable to bend, losing its pliable, willow-like quality. In severe cases there may be spasms and cramps, and these symptoms may be very sudden and violent.

'The liver channel enmeshes the genitals'

The main liver channel travels from the centre of the big toe up the inside of the leg to the groin and circles around the genitals. In women this stresses the link of the liver with menstruation and also with the muscular release in the perineum necessary for childbirth. In men it controls the erection.

The perineum is the root of muscular control for the whole body, and the gathering of the strength of the muscles in this area is called by the Chinese the 'ancestral muscle'. The male erection symbolises the effect of muscular strength and the attributes of the liver energy in its ability to rise up with life and vitality. It also graphically shows the part played by the blood in the ability of muscles to move and expand.

'The liver is averse to wind'

Wind stirs the yang of the liver, and as a yang organ amongst the organs of storage, its tendency is towards upward movement and agitation. As with the heart, too much stimulation damages the yin of the liver, ultimately depleting the blood.

Wind may be external, in the form of draughts, creating aches and pains or spasms in the muscles, or sudden changes in weather which attack the body's defence systems. It is said that any pathogen coupled with wind will enter the body more quickly and efficiently. Internal wind is created within the body by a lack of liver blood or from emotional causes, particularly suppressed anger. This kind of internal liver wind may give rise to trembling and shaking in the limbs, or headaches, blurred vision or vertigo.

'Liver depression may transform into fire'

If the depression or repression of the natural flow of the energy of the liver is continual it may transform into fire. In the cycle of generation of the five elements, wood transforms into fire, and this pattern may resemble the movement of two sticks being rubbed together. The repression of any emotion will affect the freeflow of the liver, and if the liver's natural tendency for freeflow is obstructed for too long it will flare up as severe migraine-type headaches, often with visual disturbance and noises in the ears, or in muscle spasms, convulsions and strokes.

These violent symptoms usually result from a combination of long-term factors. Heat and wind within the body may be compounded by heating and moving foods, alcohol being the most obvious. Greasy and spicy foods also activate the yang of the liver and heat the blood. Violent wind and heat damages the yin and the fluids of the body, which may then cause spasms and cramps in the muscles.

'Liver qi flows to the eyes'

Good vision again depends on the ability of the liver meridian to bring its energy and nutrition to the eyes, and an insufficiency of the yin of the liver will cause dry eyes, blurred vision and night blindness. As the mouth, the orifice of the spleen, gives the ability to distinguish the five tastes, the eyes give the ability to distinguish the five colours. By extension it is the energy of the liver which is said to give the ability to grasp that which is far away. It is an extension of the outward movement of the liver that gives the ability to see at a distance, and to have clarity of vision, on a mental as well as a physical level. It is the energy of the liver which allows us to project into the future, to make plans and decisions.

'The liver is connected to the gall-bladder'

The liver and gall-bladder have an intimate relationship, both being governed by the wood element. The gall-bladder meridian, which zigzags over the side of the head, is said to be the channel for the rising energy of the liver, and many of the symptoms of liver wind and aggressive liver energy are very closely connected with this gall-bladder pathway. Migraine headaches, for example, often follow the pathway of this meridian, over the temple and into the eyes. In terms of the emotions, the liver is often said to project plans, the gall-bladder to have the precision and ability to put them into practice. These two functions are very closely interwoven in Chinese medicine.

'The lungs govern the qi'

Qi is breath, and the lungs govern the qi of the whole body. It is through the lungs that the 'breaths of heaven' circulate, the rhythm of the lungs giving movement and circulation to the qi of the whole body. The lung meridian is the starting-point of the circulation of the 12 main meridians. Welling up from the centre of the abdomen, it surfaces on the chest and begins the circulation of energy throughout the body. It is this function of the lungs in governing qi, and the close association of qi and breath that explains the vital importance of breathing exercises in Eastern medical traditions. Therapeutic exercise depends for its effect on the use of the breath, the ability for the mind to direct the breath, and the correct combination of physical movement, breath and mental concentration.

As stillness is beneficial for the heart, and movement for the liver, so rhythmical breathing is beneficial for the lungs. All lung problems may be helped by attention to the breath. The lungs naturally expand and diffuse the breath, but it is also their function to condense and send energy down to the depths of the body. As vapours rise upwards in the body, the lungs act as a kind of 'canopy' diffusing and creating liquids that permeate the flesh and skin. In this way the lungs and the breath activate the generation of vapours and liquids in much the same way as rains are produced on the earth.

'The lung masters the nose'

This connection is very obvious. The nose is the orifice through which the 'clear' breath enters the lungs and through which the 'unclear' breath is expelled. If the nose is blocked, it is difficult for the lungs to function effectively, but Chinese medicine would also assume that the problem with the nose stems from a weakness in the energy of the lungs.

'The lungs govern the voice'

The strength and clarity of the voice show the state of the lung energy. A good loud voice shows strong lung qi, a quiet, timid voice suggests a weakness of lung qi. The strength of the voice often accompanies good posture and an open chest which allows the energy of the lungs to expand and circulate. Drooped shoulders and a sunken chest will create difficulty with the breath and eventually lung problems, and the voice tends to lack clarity and strength.

'The lungs are averse to cold'

We have all experienced the effect of cold on the lungs, and it is the sudden change of temperature in the autumn, the season of metal and the lungs, that brings most common lung problems, from colds and flus to bronchitis and pneumonia. It is the movement from the expansion of energy in the summer to the contracting and inward movement of autumn and winter that is made by the metal element and the lungs. If the metal energy is unable to contract and condense, then the body is left open to attack by the cold. This autumnal movement of withdrawl is the most difficult for us to achieve, and it is often the time when many of us get sick and depressed. We tend to enjoy the yang seasons of expansion and growth at the expense of the yin seasons of preservation and concentration, but it is important that we learn to appreciate autumn and to allow the protective movement of withdrawal to the interior that should naturally protect us at this vulnerable time of year.

'The lungs govern the skin and (body) hair'

The skin is the outward extent of the diffusion of the lung energy. Taking this further, the skin is also the connection between the lungs and the outside, and the lungs are said to govern the opening and closing of the pores, one way that wind and cold may enter the body. In the same way that perverse energy may enter the body through the pores of the skin, the body qi and essence may be lost through the pores. The closing of the pores therefore gives defence from the external influences of cold, wind, heat and damp, and protection from within by limiting the loss of essences through sweating.

As the blood and qi of the liver nourishes the muscles and tendons, the qi and fluids of the lungs nourish the skin. If the lungs are deficient in fluids, the skin will often be dry and flaky; if there is heat in the lungs there may be redness on the skin; if there is dampness, the skin may be weepy and pusy. These simple correlations help the practitioner to diagnose the particular cause of various skin problems, and adds to the success of Chinese medicine in treating skin diseases.

'The lung is connected to the large intestine'

The connection of these paired organs within the metal element is one of the more difficult to grasp, as there is no obvious link between the lungs and the large intestine in Western medicine. But the function related to metal and autumn of condensation and integration of what is useful and the letting go of all that is no longer useful for our growth can also be applied to the function of the large intestine which allows the final reabsorption of any useful elements of food and drink before letting them go. Many parallels can be drawn between a well functioning large intestine and the ability to let go of the old worn-out elements of our lives. A weak metal element may often be seen as the inability to let go.

Table 3: The Resonances of the Five Elements

	Fire	Water	Wood	Metal	Earth
Yin organ:	Heart	Kidneys	Liver	Lungs	Spleen
Yang organ:	Small Intestine	Bladder	Gall-bladder	Large intestine	Stomach
Body system:	Blood circulation	Bones and marrow	Muscles and tendons	Skin	Flesh
Orifice:	Tongue	Lower orifices	Eyes	Nose	Mouth
Taste:	Bitter	Salty	Acid	Pungent	Sweet
Governs:	Spirit	Essence	Freeflow	Qi	Transformation

THE EMOTIONS

The movements associated with the four seasons and the five elements are seen most clearly in the emotions. From the classical Chinese medical viewpoint, the emotions are merely movements of energy and, if allowed free expression, are a natural and essential part of health. It is only when they are blocked or repressed that they tend to create problems. The emotions are considered to be of equal value, no judgements being made that anger, for example, is negative, or joy positive; it is more their appropriateness at a given time. Grief is the appropriate emotion in times of bereavement, but if this emotion continues for a long time after the event, it may become pathological. Similarly, anger should be expressed at the appropriate times, but when life is lived with a constant underlying anger or a constant repression of anger, there will soon be energetic and physical symptoms.

This necessity for freeflow of the emotions automatically links the emotions to the function of the liver, and it is said that the liver is especially damaged if emotions are not expressed. But each emotion is also associated with a particular organ according to its energetic movement. The five basic emotions, joy, fear, anger, sorrow and worry relate to the five internal organs, and each organ also has its related 'virtue' – the positive influence to help balance the emotions. These are ritual, wisdom, humanity, justice and truth.

'Joy is the emotion of the heart'

Joy is the emotion that allows the spirit to move upwards. If the heart is calm there is a peaceful joy that permeates the whole being. It is a calm, detached sense of the self at peace with the world, which is beneficial for the heart and for all the organs. It is also a centredness that allows the other emotions to come and go without attachment. It is the joy of being alive. In excess, there may be an ecstatic, excitable joy, scattering the spirits in its exaggerated upward movement and losing anchorage in common sense. The natural uplifting of the heart energy becomes almost manic, and the shine of the spirit in the eyes is too bright.

The classical Chinese texts use two characters for joy, one for this deeper, centred sense of self, the other for excitement and elation, and both characters have their root in types of music. The first relates to the ceremonial music, played during certain rites, that gives balance and draws people together in harmony, the other to a kind of drum music played for dancing at popular feasts and celebrations.

The 'virtue' of the heart is said to be ritual. In ancient times, ritual created a way to be in touch with the spirit, creating inner joy and providing an expression for ecstatic joy, raising up the heart and creating space and openness in the chest.

Western society has abolished much of its ritual, which in the past has provided nourishment for the soul. Without this nourishment, we often develop a deep longing that may surface in various ways as cravings and addictions. We crave excitement and external stimulation to keep the heart uplifted, and more and more we tend to rely on external factors for our happiness in a kind of addiction to joy. We get hooked on food, alcohol, drugs or shopping to satiate our inner cravings, our personal addiction tending to follow the patterns of our own particular energetic imbalance.

We decided to discard our old rituals as they no longer spoke to our souls, but we have not yet found a replacement. We are in a time of flux, a society in search of new rituals, the society of the shopping mall. It has been suggested that the rave culture is an attempt by youth to create their own rituals, their own heart-centred ecstatic tribal dance. And perhaps this is just another sign that we are beginning to incorporate the wisdom of the ancient earth-based religions back into our soulless societies.

'The emotion of the kidneys is fear'

Fear is linked to the cold, to the dark, to the night, to the winter. The fear of the kidneys is a fear for our survival, at an animal and instinctive level. Fear is related to cold as joy is related to warmth. We shiver from fear and we shiver from cold. It is the emotion that causes the energy to descend.

The Chinese medical classics describe fear as causing a blockage in the circulation between the upper part of the body (the heart) and the lower (the kidneys), causing agitation in the heart, and a loss of the retentive power of the kidneys. If this lower centre cannot retain, energy will drain away downwards; in acute states of fear the lower orifices cannot hold, and common expressions like being 'shit scared' are familiar to us all. Long-term fear can create a separation of yin and yang in the lower abdomen and a leakage of essences through the lower orifices in spermatorrhea, leucorrhea and certain kinds of chronic diarrhoea.

In the same way that joy is not always seen as a positive emotion, fear is not always negative. Our fears are the areas of our life we must deal with in order to grow and develop emotionally, and by facing our fears we evolve will and wisdom. Also associated with the kidneys and the water element are the kind of stability and common sense that come from this grounding in reality, a healthy caution that can counteract excessive joy or elation.

Wisdom is the 'virtue' of the kidneys and is a practical kind of know-how, a *savoir-faire*, the ability to act and get things done as much as to know the correct thing to do. It is a grounded and earthed wisdom which is based in the will to live, and on the reality of circumstances.

'Anger is the emotion of the liver'

We touched on the association of anger with the liver when we discussed 'freeflow'. Energetically, anger moves upwards and outwards. Its movement is similar to that of joy, and we have seen before that the heart and the liver both have this yang upward movement. But unlike the joy of the heart, which even in imbalance is about being 'high', there is much more force and violence associated with anger. The energy of wood, the wind and of spring are all violent and sudden. It is the energy associated with birth and the natural violence of all beginnings of life. It is a powerforce that is often likened to the release of an arrow from a bow, or a coiled spring released. It is the power of life to burst through the frozen earth in the springtime.

Similarly, anger at the appropriate time can have a creative power to release blockages, give direction to life, to stimulate and move forward. But if this natural life force is blocked, it can created havoc in the body, giving rise to all kinds of violent symptoms, from migraines to strokes.

Anger should be expressed and released, never held on to or blocked. But we must always be careful to know if our anger is appropriate. If it becomes our usual response in difficult situations, possibly the upward/outward impulse is not allowing inner reflection and a natural freeflow between ourselves and others. The 'virtue' of the liver and the wood element is humanity; the ability to relate naturally and humanely to others. It is to treat others as we would have them treat us, to walk in their shoes, to have compassion. And if we develop compassion there is little need for anger, except where it is appropriate.

'Sorrow is the emotion of the lungs'

Sorrow relates to the autumn and it is the movement of compression, depression, oppression and deflation. Autumn is often the most difficult time of year as it is the transition from openness and expansion to construction and introspection. In the cycle of the five elements this transition is aided by the element earth, which governs late summer and harvest.

All cultures view the autumn as the time of judgement, of balancing the scales. It is a time of letting go, as trees let go of their leaves, to conserve energy for the winter. And psychologically, this is the time for seeing things as they really are, getting rid of what is not essential and preparing for the descent into the underworld. Pathologically, this sadness that is connected to the movement of autumn is the inability to accept the reality of life, and it is a movement inwards which contracts the energy channels around the heart; the chest becomes sunken and the shoulders rounded.

Sadness and grief are appropriate when there is loss; there is an inability to believe in the reality of the situation, which is natural, but if this continues for too long then it becomes pathological, causing blockage in the chest and lungs. Many cases of asthma in adults can be traced to a time of grief, the loss of a partner or a parent where there was either a descent into grief and sadness which proved impossible to climb out of, or the inability to grieve; both are a different kind of powerlessness to accept what is.

Here again the lack of ritual in our lives denies us the space and time to allow our emotions to readjust to a new reality. Around death we are expected to carry on as if nothing has happened. Our culture attempts to make light of death because we do not know how to deal with it. Death has lost its place in our lives, and therefore we do not know how to grieve.

Exercises to open the chest and stimulate the lungs – to open the body to an influx of new life and vitality – are often the most effective way to counteract the action of sadness and grief and its effects on the lungs. Deep breathing, walking, moving, stretching, massaging the back and shoulders all relieve the tightness around the heart. Once the body begins to open and energy begins to flow the oppression is released and the spirits begin to rise. The difficulty is making the first steps, and many people need help and encouragement.

The virtue of the lungs is justice, which in its pure form is nothing other than the ability to see things as they really are.

'The emotion of the spleen is thought'

The energy of the spleen allows the ability to turn things over in the mind, to reflect, to consider. It is quite difficult to understand thought as a negative emotion without reference to the earth and to its associated movement of continual turning and churning. If this movement in the psyche is extreme it can become worry and concern.

The earth has the ability to discern what is of value and what is not of value, and in the same way that the spleen takes in food and distinguishes the pure and the impure, the earth energy in the emotional realm takes in information and sifts what is of value and what is not of value. It gives discernment, both in food for the body and food for the mind.

The pathological emotion associated with the spleen is usually translated as obsessive thought. When thoughts go round and round with no direction they create knots which block energy flow. There is lack of transformation and transportation, creating blockage in the centre. The Chinese medical classics tell us that 'anger dominates obsessive thought', and a violent surge of energy is often what is needed to break through this kind of stuckness, to make a decision and to move forward. The knotting of energy in the centre, which can often be felt as a constriction above the navel, under the ribcage, will upset the communication between the heart and the kidneys, eventually causing insomnia and even fear. If obsessive thought continues, it is said to 'scatter the purpose' and create desire – the desire to possess things, people, and to control.

The 'virtue' of the spleen is truth and loyalty or, more literally, the effect of one's words on another.

Fright

The emotion of fright, or starting with fright, which is often mentioned in the Chinese medical texts, is not associated with one particular organ but with the relationship between the heart and the kidneys or the liver and kidneys. It is a kind of jumpiness, and may manifest in starting at sudden noises or waking suddenly and easily from sleep; the etymology of the Chinese character suggests a temperamental horse, reacting at the slightest change.

If the jumpiness is muscular it suggests a connection with the liver, possibly a lack of liver blood and a consequent failure to nourish the muscles. If there are palpitations there is more likely to be a connection with the heart and a lack of control of the descending power of the kidneys on the ascending power of the heart. The kidneys root the energy, especially at night, and any jumpiness during the night would be related to the inability of the kidneys to hold the energy down. This is usually seen as a lack of relationship between the heart and the kidneys, or the spirit and will, and often occurs when extreme stress has depleted both the yin and the yang, causing them to pull apart. In extreme cases fright can cause muscle spasms and fits, and in China it is often claimed that if a pregnant woman experiences a great fright it can cause fits in her baby from birth.

Oppression

Oppression is usually listed as the seventh emotion, and although this particularly affects the heart, it may be seen wherever there is an obstruction to the natural movement of qi.

Most pathological emotions come from the inability to accept the nature and circumstances of life. The ability to adapt and change is therefore seen as the most important factor in mental as well as physical health. There must always be balance, and we read in the medical classics that fear dominates elation and grief dominates anger; the vitality of life can break through sadness, and joy can overcome our deepest fears.

THE SPIRITS

The translation of the Chinese terms for the spiritual aspects associated with the five elements and the five internal organs have caused difficulty for translators over the years. They have been the source of much confusion, not just because we do not have the appropriate words but because the concepts themselves are difficult to grasp. The Chinese term for spirit, shen, can be translated as spirit, mind or consciousness. The history of Chinese medicine is long, and it is not surprising that there have been many different ways of looking at 'spirit' over the centuries; it would be much the same in any culture. But certainly in the days of the oldest medical texts, shen would have been translated in the plural, suggesting a multitude of spirits or benign influences from heaven.

In the same way that the sun is always in the sky but can be obscured by clouds, so the heavenly influence of the shen is always present, but may be obscured from us by clouds of negative emotion. These clouds may manifest on a spiritual, mental, emotional or physical level. If we create a particular 'anger cloud', we may expect to feel effects on the physical level along the resonances of the liver with, for example, headaches or menstrual problems, or as a disturbance of the spirit of the liver with excess dreaming, or, in an extreme case, with involuntary astral projection.

Thus the physical, emotional and spiritual aspects are seen as a continuum, and intervention at any level may redress imbalance and restore health. *The Yellow Emperor's Classic of Internal Medicine* tells us that unless we treat the root (of the illness) we will not reach the spirits, and unless every level is taken into consideration there may not be a permanent cure. If we diagnose and treat a menstrual disorder without taking into consideration anger and irritability, we may achieve a temporary cure, but the symptoms are likely to re-emerge in time.

The term shen is used collectively for the spiritual aspects of all the organs, and also specifically as the spirit linked with the heart. As the heart is the 'emperor' in the physical realm, so the spirits of the heart govern the spiritual and psychic realms. Each of the organs has its presiding spirit, and these spirits are guided by the shen. The shen of the heart is most ethereal, the liver slightly less so, until we reach the spirit of the lungs which belongs more to the body and the earth. These spirits create a kind of field of consciousness which allows the various physical aspects to manifest in a particular way. They could be described as the guiding principles of life, which oversee the transformation of matter into a living being.

The shen are responsible for individuality, for psychic and mental faculties, but are also present in every part of the physical body, bringing intelligence to the cells.

'The heart stores the spirit (shen)'

We discussed the heart and its relation to spirit earlier, and in Chinese medicine it is impossible to speak of the heart without its connection with the spirits. All heart pathology is a 'clouding of the spirits'. The image of clouds in the sky is often used to describe the need for clarity and emptiness in the human heart; a clarity of mind and calmness within the body which allows the spirits to shine, and which allows the natural intelligence of the body to work unimpeded. The spirit of the heart works with the spirit of the spleen to attain discernment, with the spirit of the liver to attain vision and the ability to move forward and plan, with the spirit of the lungs to maintain the bodily rhythms and with the spirit of the kidneys to develop strength and a deep understanding of life.

'The liver stores the hun (soul)'

In classical texts the hun are said to come and go with the spirits, shen. We have seen many times in our discussion of the organs that the heart and liver share similar energetics, and it is again this upward, outward movement that unites the shen and hun. Many translators call the shen the universal spirit and the hun the individual human soul, the aspect of the shen embodied within the individual.

The liver has the ability to expand, to move, to project, to see into the distance, and all these attributes are made possible by the hun. The hun allow dreams, imagination, clairvoyance, astral projections – and at the same time they depend upon the blood of the liver to hold them, to stop them floating away. The blood, the yin aspect of the liver, gives the hun a firm base from which to project, to follow the pure spirit, but always to come back to the body. If the blood is weak, the hun may fly off and have difficulty returning; the body may continue to function, but the consciousness is no longer there.

During deep meditation, the hun may be far away, leaving the body in a state of suspended animation, no longer able to speak, to see or to hear, but functioning perfectly on an autonomic level. Chinese alchemy tells us that there are three hun, one in each of the three energetic centres, or dan tian, situated below the navel, at the centre of the chest, and between the eyebrows. These three centres correspond in the Indian chakra system to the swadhisthana, the anahata and the ajna chakras. Excessive dreaming and even involuntary astral projection may be due to a lack of liver blood, and could be treated with various blood and yin tonics. In Chinese herbal medicine, minerals are often used to control an over-active hun, their very weight and substance being used to anchor the floating hun.

'The lungs store the po (the bodily soul)'

As the spirits are balanced by the essences, so the hun are balanced by the po. The po are sometimes called the animal soul, or the corporeal soul, but may be best understood as the intelligence that remains when the hun are not there. It is the autonomic regulation that keeps the lungs inhaling and exhaling, the heart beating, the digestive system transforming and transporting in the state of deep meditation or coma. Their relationship to the lungs becomes clearer when we understand that it is the rhythm of the breath that gives the rhythm and impulse for all these instinctive functions. By controlling the breath it is possible to slow down the bodily functions until there is a state of near hibernation, and many Indian yogis have been known to slow their heart rate and their metabolism by control of the breath.

The lack of this essential rhythm can be seen in some cases of Chronic Fatigue Syndrome, where the body virtually forgets how to breathe. All the bodily functions which we take so much for granted begin to break down, the rhythms of sleep, the ability to process and absorb nourishment from food, even the beating of the heart begin to act in a random way. A new rhythm must be consciously relearnt, and simple breathing exercises are very effective if practised consistently.

The po organise the essences, the structure, the movement of gathering in and collecting that is peculiar to the metal element and to yin. As the hun relate to the liver and depend for their function on the liver blood, so the po relate to the lungs and rely on the qi for their distribution.

'The spleen stores the purpose (yi)'

Being connected with the spleen and the earth, the purpose, yi, represents the centre, and especially that which harmoniously balances the spirits resting in the heart and the will centred in the kidneys. The purpose mediates that which comes from the outside world. As the spleen facilitates the absorption of food from the external world and allows it to be incorporated into the body, so the purpose allows the incorporation of mental and psychic energies. And as the spleen must discern good and bad food through the five tastes, the purpose must be able to discern good and bad ideas and psychic influences.

The Chinese character for yi is made up of a muscial note and the character for heart, thus the purpose must be in resonance with the heart to be able to discern what to accept from the outside. When an idea resonates with the heart it is said to create purpose – when purpose is held it becomes will.

In pathology, a weakness of the yi may result in lack of discernment as regards ideas and psychic influences. According to the Indian tradition, energy may enter and leave the body most easily through the centre related to the spleen and stomach, and it is vital to guard against intrusion of undesirable psychic forces. Involuntary psychic possession is most likely to occur through the spleen centre, and must involve a lack of yi.

'The kidneys store the will (zhi)'

The will, which is stored in the kidneys, is a deep evolutionary urge, a push for the individual to fulfil his or her unique potential. On a more mundane level it is the will to live, the will to survive, the will to continue the species, the sex drive, an energy which in most spiritual traditions and in many different ways can be transformed from a basic reproductive urge to a means of spiritual growth. Its relationship, via the kidneys, to the lower parts of the trunk, to the spine and to the brain make it impossible not to draw parallels with the Indian concept of kundalini, which, from its seat at the base of the spine, inspires the transformation and transmutation of evolutionary energies.

The kidneys always represent a balance of yin and yang characteristics, and as we saw earlier in the relationship of the bones and the marrow, the teeth and the hair, the hard and the soft are also contrasted in describing the will. The will must be strong, but it must not be fixed. If it is unable to adapt, it is weak. In martial arts, which stress the strength of the kidneys and lower abdomen, strength often comes through the ability to change and flow. So the will must be strong, but it must also be supple. Pathologically, a lack of will may create addictive patterns of behaviour, most obviously sexual addictions, but equally those of addiction to romance, alcohol, drugs – in fact anything that ultimately sidetracks our growth and development.

It is the balance of these five spiritual aspects that brings physical, emotional and spiritual health, not the cultivation of one at the expense of the other. There is no sense in Chinese thought of spirit and matter in conflict, and even the most spiritual disciplines of Daoist yoga stress the importance of maintaining the physical body. Some practices aim at the immortality of the body rather than the afterlife. All is in the balance of the earthly and heavenly energies, matter and spirit, yin and yang.

Table 4: The Emotions and Spirits

	Fire	Water	Wood	Metal	Earth
Organ:	Heart	Kidneys	Liver	Lungs	Spleen
Emotion:	Joy	Fear	Anger	Sadness	Overthinking
Spiritual aspect:	Spirit, shen	Will, zhi	Soul, hun	Bodily soul, po	Purpose, yi
Virtue:	Ritual	Wisdom	Humanity	Justice	Truth
Focus:	Aspiration	Grounding	Imagination	Letting go	Centredness

PART 2

THE BODILY LANDSCAPE

Learning about Energy Flow

The information in this section aims to give a basic understanding of the Chinese view of the subtle energy body. We will begin with a description of the meridian system, looking briefly at the 12 main meridians, which are linked to the five elements and the internal organs, before progressing to the eight extraordinary meridians, which form the basis for qi gong and meditation practice. There is much new information and the concepts and terminology may be difficult to grasp at first, but although highly complex in its detail of points and interconnections, the basis of the meridian system remains simple – the yin meridians flow upwards from the earth bringing nourishment and grounding, the yang meridians flow downwards from heaven bringing movement and vitality. By remembering this and applying it in massage and exercise we can do much towards our self-healing.

The language traditionally used to describe the bodily landscape is often symbolic and poetic – and many translators of Daoist alchemical texts have assumed it to be deliberately obscure. But the names of acupuncture points, for example, which often include terms such as well, spring, pool or sea, can give a graphic description of the energy flow at a particular location on the body. It is certainly not necessary to understand the name of an acupuncture point for it to be effective; a name is useful only if it helps you to understand the energy behind the words – but a basic understanding of this system of energy channels enables us to comprehend the otherwise mystifying field of Oriental exercise and self-massage. So much confusion arises because the movement has been divorced from its root; if you can begin to picture what you are doing and why, actions have a far greater potency.

Work with the information and meditate on it, a bit at a time. Allow these ideas to seep into your consciousness as you perform the exercises and visualisations. Don't struggle with it. They are presented as an aid but should not become an obstacle. You may find it most beneficial to use this section as reference for the exercise and massage techniques described in Parts 3, 4 and 5.

The concept of subtle energies exists in most cultures; many share a similar idea of energy centres, fewer have a concept of subtle energy channels. The Indian and the Chinese views of the energy body are exceptional in that they have been incorporated into the traditional medicine rather than remaining in the realms of the esoteric, and have therefore developed in detail and intricacy. The Chinese system of the acupuncture meridians and their specific points of influence is probably the most highly developed and the cross-fertilisation of ideas throughout Tibet, China and South-east Asia has provided a rich diversity of this tradition. The Chinese vision of the bodily landscape was imported into Japan where it has flourished and grown, both within medicine and the disciplines of meditation and the martial arts.

The Chinese meridian system has similarities with the Indian concept of chakras and nadis, but the Chinese have been more concerned with the physical realms, the Indian culture with the spiritual. The Chinese directed their knowledge more towards medicine, and even in their spiritual practice were more concerned with immortality than the afterlife, considering good health to go hand in hand with spiritual realisation. The Indian spiritual tradition, on the other hand, has often stressed the transcendence of the body, some schools believing that the body should be virtually tortured in order to obtain liberation of the soul. Because of this ancient preoccupation with health and longevity, it is within the Chinese system that we find the most practical and highly developed descriptions of the pathways of subtle energy within the body.

Scientists in the East and the West investigating the effects of acupuncture are trying to rationalise subtle energy flow in terms of the logical, the provable. The fact that they are often unsuccessful may prove to be a shortcoming of their scientific methodology rather than of the system itself. Much is already known and accepted of the non-physical in certain areas of theoretical physics, but the medical profession is practically based and resistant to change; the drug companies are a powerful force to keep things as they are. However, the acceptance and understanding of these subtle energies will prove vital in the medicine of the future.

Western medical science has attempted to explain the effects of acupuncture by nerve pathways, chemical triggers, and these mechanisms certainly play their part in the thera-peutic effect, particularly in pain relief. But in order to understand the more complex effects of acupuncture, and of Oriental exercise and massage, an acceptance of the meridian system, or system of energetic transference, is essential, as it is the premise on which they are based. Science is making great progress in naming the unnameable and seeing the invisible – and soon scientists may be able to make their own maps of the bodily landscape. But in the meantime the most effective way to make this irrational information accessible and acceptable to the mind is to experience it within the body.

Many times within an acupuncture treatment a patient will describe a sensation along a channel without any previous knowledge of the pathway. And diverse groups of symptoms are often seen to be interlinked when looked at in the light of the meridian system. Our bodies respond to this kind of information. The first time I went for an acupuncture treat-ment in Japan, the pathway of my imbalanced meridian was pointed out on a wall chart. The pathway of the meridian corresponded to the pain of my headaches, and the related area of the spine to a recent back injury. The information immediately made sense to my body even though I had no idea how to file it away in my mind. It was one of those bits of information that have to wait patiently until a bigger world view can be achieved.

THE TWELVE MAIN MERIDIANS

Chinese philosophy suggests that all life exists through an energetic interchange of the powers of heaven and earth. The light, animating energy of heaven, heavenly qi, mingles with the heavier, dense energy of earth to create all life. At this level there is no distinction between energy and matter – matter is seen as a slower vibration, a denser version of the same basic energy which underlies and animates all things. The way in which this energy, or qi, intermingles, the patterns that are followed, determines the life forms that evolve. The earth has its own energetic laws which are studied by the Chinese in the science of feng shui, or Chinese geomancy. The earth has its hills and valleys, rivers and seas, and each place creates its own energetic tendency, whether damp and boggy, fresh and windy, dry and arid. The ancient medical texts describe the bodily landscape in similar terms, and see the body as made up of ravines and valleys, plains and seas; the names of acupuncture points often reflect this poetic terminology.

Plants draw their nourishment from the earth and their transformative power from the sun, conforming to the regulation of the four seasons in their growth and flowering, their shedding and their seeding. In the same way the energies of heaven and earth intermingle within the body of humankind. And as the earth has its own energy pattern or energy grids, so the human body has a similar network of energy pathways – quite complex and intricate, but always based upon the simple idea that the yin earth energy travels upwards from the feet, through the legs and into the abdomen and chest, the yang heavenly energy travels down through the head and the hands towards the feet (see Plate 1).

The meridian system has three main yang pathways and three main yin pathways, which are subdivided into an arm and a leg meridian. There are therefore a total of 12 main meridians which traverse the surface of the body and each one is related to an internal organ. Each meridian has an identical pathway on the left and the right of the body, creating a mirror image of left and right.

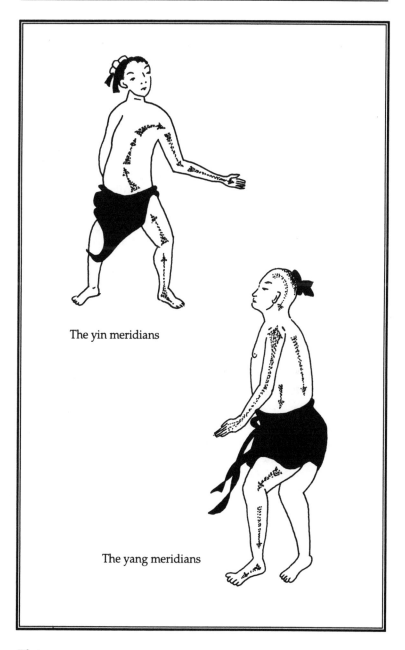

The yin meridians

The yang meridians

Plate 1

The yin meridians related to the spleen, liver and kidneys begin in the feet and travel up the inside of the legs into the lower abdomen where they bind together before spreading over the abdomen and into the chest. In the chest they link with the three yin meridians of the arms; the kidney meridian links with the heart, the spleen meridian with the lungs, and the liver with the heart master, the second meridian related to the heart (see Plate 2).

The spleen and lungs form the tai yin or great yin meridian, the kidneys and heart the shao yin or lesser yin meridian, the liver and heart master the jue yin or extreme yin meridian. The arm yin meridians flow from the chest along the inside of the arm, across the palm of the hand to the fingertips.

The heart has two meridians, one associated with the heart as the seat of the spirit and the emotions, the other, the heart master, or recently called the pericardium, more concerned with the physiological heart. In the classical texts, the meridian of the heart itself is rarely treated and in certain texts it is not mentioned at all. It was possibly considered too dangerous to interfere with the energy of the spirit.

If we stand with our arms above the head, the yin meridians make one movement up through the body, drawing energy from the earth through the soles of the feet, binding round the ankles, up the inside of the calf, around the inner knee and up the inner thigh to the groin, where the liver meridian binds around the genitals. All three yin meridians of the legs meet together in the lower abdomen, spread up into the chest where they continue up through the armpit and up the inside of the arms, penetrating the wrists and flowing to the fingertips, the lighter energy of the heart and lungs making contact with heaven.

The yang meridians of the large intestine, the small intestine and the triple heater flow through the fingertips along the outside of the arm, into the shoulders, through the neck and into the head. The triple heater meridian is not associated with a particular organ, but with the general function of metabolism and energy production, as we shall see later. These three meridians connect with the yang meridians of the bladder, the gall-bladder and the stomach around the eyes

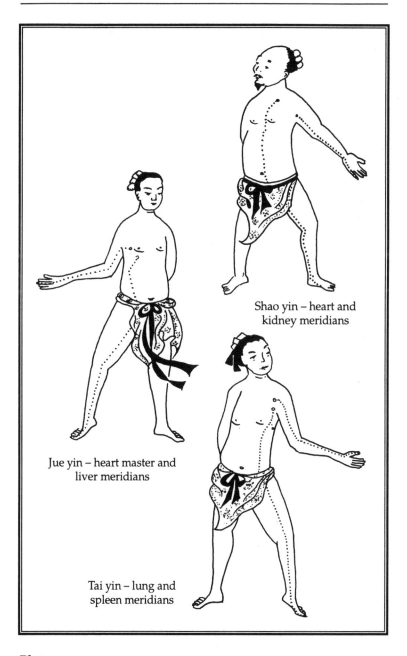

Shao yin – heart and
kidney meridians

Jue yin – heart master and
liver meridians

Tai yin – lung and
spleen meridians

Plate 2

and flow downwards. The bladder meridian flows bilaterally over the top of the head and follows either side of the spine down the back of the legs into the feet; the gall-bladder meridian flows over the sides of the head, around the shoulders and down the sides of the trunk and legs into the feet; the stomach meridian, from under the eye, down the centre of the cheeks and through the front of the body, over the nipples, into the groin and down the front of the legs and the top of the feet into the toes (see Plate 3).

The small intestine and the bladder, having the longest pathway, are called the tai yang, or great yang. The stomach and large intestine are called the yang ming, or bright yang; the triple heater and gall-bladder the shao yang, or lesser yang.

As well as their superficial pathways these 12 main meridians also have a network of interconnections and deep pathways which link each meridian with its associated organ and orifice, and make connections between yin and yang associated meridians and organs. For example, the liver meridian links with both the liver and gall-bladder organ, has many interconnections with the gall-bladder meridian and a deep pathway to its associated orifice, the eye. In the same way, a deep pathway of the heart meridian connects with the root of the tongue, and the heart meridian is often treated in loss of voice, especially due to shock. Shock is said to block the energy of the heart, and this blockage literally stops the movement of the tongue.

These 12 main meridians have particular points or, more precisely, hollows, which are treated by the acupuncturist and also used in finger pressure and massage. Points on each meridian can be used both to balance the energy of the associated element or for a more specific function related to its internal pathways and interconnections. Classically 365 points are counted along the channels, but of these 365 a small repertoire of basic points is all that is necessary for successful home treatment. In Parts 3, 4 and 5 we will look again at these 12 meridians and get to know a few of their most effective points.

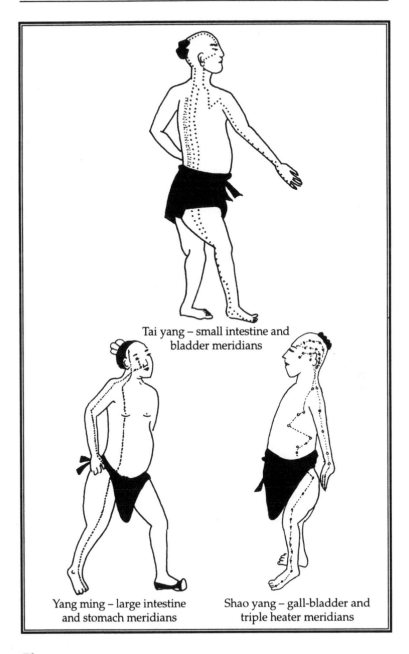

Tai yang – small intestine and
bladder meridians

Yang ming – large intestine
and stomach meridians

Shao yang – gall-bladder and
triple heater meridians

Plate 3

THE EIGHT EXTRAORDINARY MERIDIANS

Behind the complexity of the 12 meridians, with all their points and interconnections, lies an older, more basic network of pathways. They are the eight extraordinary meridians, and an understanding of their function provides a foundation for the Chinese concept of the energy body. These eight meridians ensure the basic balance of energy within the yin and the yang, the top and the bottom, the left and the right, the interior and the exterior. And it is the attainment of balance and harmony of the functions governed by these meridians that is the aim of many Daoist meditational practices and qi gong exercise.

The eight extraordinary meridians have a deeper, more primitive nature than the 12 ordinary meridians and are responsible for much of our growth and development. They carry our inherited tendencies and possibly contain the seeds of karmic illness. Whereas the 12 ordinary meridians gradually develop their functions as the body matures through the processes of crawling, standing and walking, the eight extraordinary meridians are developing within the body from the moment of conception. They are responsible for the primitive organisation of the developing embryo, from the first cell division to the perfected and fully functional organism. These eight extraordinary meridians could be said to create a kind of energy field within which the embryo develops. At birth their functions are overtaken by the 12 ordinary meridians, but they remain behind and beneath all the more diverse and complex actions of the 12, providing a reminder of a basic pattern of symmetry and wholeness.

As we grow and develop, experience trauma and illness, undergo operations and emotional upsets, the symmetry and wholeness of our bodily landscape is lost. We get dented here, scarred there, hunched up on the left, weakened on the right. Many alternative practitioners working with subtle energies see their task as being to recreate our original energetic symmetry, to get rid of blocks, to heal scars and restore a healthy energy flow. Whether we are using needles, touch, visualisation or movement, this is the aim of our treatment.

Numerology is important in understanding Chinese medicine, and it is significant here that there are eight meridians. Each number has its ancient symbolism, and eight is the number of complete perfected space. As four is the number of the four directions, north, south, east and west, and represents space on the horizontal plane, eight relates to the eight winds which fill the three-dimensional space between heaven and earth, and the eight trigrams of the *I Ching*, which represent all possible energetic phenomena. The eight of these eight meridians suggests a perfection of energy interchange between heaven and earth.

An understanding of the functions of these eight extraordinary meridians can help us to practise exercise and meditation, visualisation and self-massage with clarity and purpose, by providing a model for the body to work with. Beginning with the first division of yin and yang, we will attempt to construct a three-dimensional model of our wholeness, introducing specific points for concentration and massage as they add to the picture, creating a landscape of our energy bodies to use with visualisation.

PRIMARY YIN AND YANG

The first pair within the eight extraordinary meridians represent the primary division between yang and yin, light and dark, soft and hard. From their joint origin in the centre of the belly they gradually differentiate in the groin and surface to run along the centre back and centre front of the body, meeting again inside the mouth. Within the foetus we can see that the back is exposed to the light, has strength and hardness and this is the area of yang. The centre front is curled up towards the interior; it is soft and is the area of the yin. The nutrition from the mother flows in through the central yin channel and the lower abdominal area is the most concentrated area of yin energy.

Only these first two of the eight meridians have specific pathways and points. The first, usually called the governor vessel or, in the Chinese, du mai, follows the spine on the back, and the second, the conception vessel or ren mai, follows the centre front, forming an interlinking circle. Daoist breathing exercises and visualisations that use these two channels are sometimes called 'embryonic breathing' and aim to create balance between yin and yang, and aid the return to symmetry and wholeness.

The governor vessel (du mai)

The governor vessel oversees the yang functions of the body. It commands the yang meridians responsible for movement, warmth and transformation. The Chinese character du which is generally translated as governor, contains the idea of the ability to rule, to take charge and to create guidelines for life. Beginning in the depths of the lower abdomen, the governor vessel flows to the surface in the perineum, its first point being between the coccyx and the anus. Its pathway follows the spinal cord and penetrates the brain at the back of the head, flowing over the top of the head between the eyebrows and into the mouth (see Plate 4).

The acupuncture meridians were given a systematic series of numbers only a few hundred years ago, and particularly in the case of the extraordinary meridians, there is no specifically directional flow. Although the meridian is usually described as beginning in the lower abdomen and rising, this is more an indication of its development than of its flow. Movement is possible in both directions along the pathway, as it is for all meridians. Modern research in Japan has suggested that the tendency for movement along these primary yin and yang channels may be different for men and for women. Dr Hiroshi Motoyama suggests that a directional flow up the spine and down the front of the body is more likely in men, whereas in women the energy is more likely to flow up the front of the body and down the spine.

Let us look at a few points along this pathway that are important in visualisation and meditation and give us an insight into the nature of the pathway.

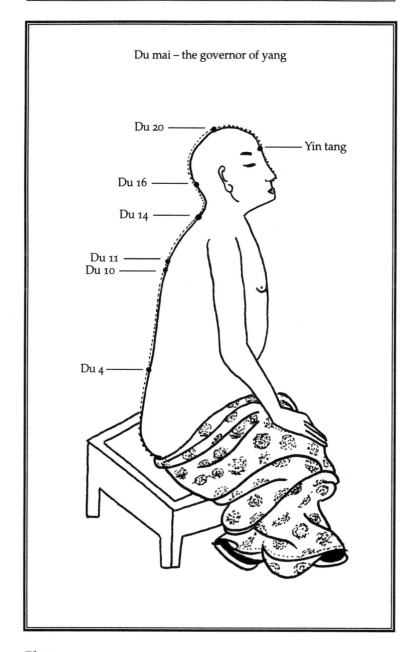

Du mai – the governor of yang

Du 20

Yin tang

Du 16

Du 14

Du 11
Du 10

Du 4

Plate 4

71

Governor vessel 1: Long and strong (chang qiang)

It is midway between the anus and the coccyx and the name of this point suggests something that is very strong and durable with the ability to provide a firm basis. For example, if the muscles in this area have a good strength and tension, they provide the strength for the body to stand straight and the organs to be held in their proper place. If the muscles are weak, there is prolapse and sagging and lack of strength in the spine.

The Chinese character qiang contains the image of an archer's bow, which is often used to illustrate the way in which energy needs to be strongly held and rooted in order to provide movement and expansion. If the bow is very firm and strong, it has the power to shoot an arrow a long distance. This dynamic tension of the bow, which is also mentioned in the function of the kidneys, is a tight, controlled holding – ready to release a surge of energy. If the base of the spine is strong enough in its holding and containing, the clear yang is able to reach the head and the brain, bringing clarity to the mind.

Focus on this point to ground the energy, to create a strong foundation. At the beginning of any exercise it is useful to be aware of this area. Contract the muscles of the perineum slightly throughout the breathing and qi gong exercises. This gives a solid base for the position and roots the breath.

Governor vessel 4: The gate of life (ming men)

This point on the spine at the level of the waist (below the 2nd lumbar vertebra) is at the same level as the main points to treat the kidney energy, and the functions of the point are strongly linked with the function of the kidneys. We have seen that the fire of the gate of life provides the energy for all transformation and transmutation within the body and the basis of metabolism and immunity. In Daoist inner alchemy this is the first stage for the transformation of coarse material substance into the finer energies. Symbolically, the gate of life is said to provide the link between your inherited energies and tendencies and your ability to transform and transmute them in order to fulfil your potential. It is your link with both your origin and your possible evolution.

This is the major point in the body for strengthening the yang, the moving, warming and vitalising energy. It can be heated with moxa in all cases of energy depletion, warmed with the hands, stretched and stimulated with exercise. It is one of the most important points on the body, and will be referred to many times in Parts 3, 4 and 5.

Governor vessel 10: Spirit watchtower (ling tai)
This point is on the spine at the level of the heart (below the 6th thoracic vertebra). The watchtower guards the heart and allows access only to pure energy. This is the first point above the diaphragm, and the diaphragm acts as a kind of filter allowing only the pure qi into the area of the heart and lungs.

In ancient times the spirit watchtower was the name given to a tower used by the emperor to observe the kingdom and also to watch the stars. By gaining important knowledge and information both of earth and heaven, he would be able to make the proper informed decisions to rule the kingdom. The heart is often called the emperor and must be able to receive all the relevant information in order to master the body. In the body, all perceptions and information have to be presented to the heart which, if it is quiet and calm, is able to discern the reality of the situation and adapt accordingly.

Governor vessel 11: The way of the spirits (shen dao)
On the spine at the level of the heart (below the 5th thoracic vertebra), this point is often referred to as the second of the three major 'stations' of the meridian, the first being the gate of life, relating to the lower energy centre, the third being the palace of impressions, between the eyebrows and relating to the upper energy centre. This point obviously relates to the heart centre and, as we have seen, the heart is said to 'store the spirit'. This same term in Japanese is Shinto, and expresses the need to live in harmony with the spirit of the universe and also with your own spirit.

In many texts governor vessel points 10 and 11 are contra-indicated for acupuncture, which suggests the sensitivity of the energy at this level. Many acupuncture points have been forbidden at different times throughout the history of Chinese medicine and by different schools. Points which strongly affect the heart are the most commonly forbidden points. 'Heart therapy' is therefore often based around breathing, meditation and visualisation techniques – all aimed to calm the heart. If the heart is calm, the spirit can be at rest.

It is important that this vital area of the spine is kept flexible and loose. Muscle tension can tighten the diaphragm and interfere with the natural flow of qi around the heart and lungs. Move your shoulders, breathe deeply, release and relax.

Governor vessel 14: Great hammer (da zhui)

The name of this point, which is at the top of the back, between the 7th cervical and 1st thoracic vertebrae, refers to the bodily landscape and the protrusion of the bones in this area. It is at the level of the shoulders, and it is here that all the yang meridians of the body meet and bind together, in much the same way as the yin meridians gather in the lower abdomen. It is the last point of the governor vessel on the trunk, and is often treated to allow freeflow of energy between the head and the body. Many neck exercises work to free tension and accumulation around this area, to loosen the neck and shoulders and release headaches.

Governor vessel 16: The storehouse of the wind (feng fu)

It is at this point, on the midline at the base of the skull, that the governor vessel has a deep pathway which enters the brain, the yang energy of the meridian bringing clarity to the brain and aiding clear thought and perception. But wind and cold can also penetrate the head around the base of the skull and it is important to protect this area from the effects of cold wind.

Tension in the neck and the base of the skull is very common, and easily results both in headache and muddled thinking. It is important to keep this area mobile with simple neck stretching exercises for the full effects of the clarity of the yang to reach the brain.

Governor vessel 20: One hundred meetings (bai hui)
This point is at the top of the head, the depression in line with the tips of the ears. It is the meeting place of the six yang meridians and the governor vessel; the apex of the head is visualised in qi gong and tai ji as the point from which the body is suspended. Get to know this important point. Take a strand of hair from around the point and pull upwards. The chin naturally tucks in and the back of the neck extends, allowing a good circulation in the neck and head.

This point is used to resuscitate the energy in all kinds of fainting and collapse, and also to treat prolapse in the lower abdomen and orifices.

The hall of the seal (yin tang)
On the midline, between the eyebrows (no number), this is the point of concentration for the brow centre, ajna chakra, or in Chinese alchemical terms, the upper dan tian. In most systems the eyebrow centre is the place of the detached, objective witness, the centre of control linked with the pituitary gland, which itself controls the other glands in the body.

It is used in Daoist meditation techniques, though rarely mentioned in medicine. It is listed as an 'extra point' in modern acupuncture books, but not as an official point of the governor vessel. We will come across it in reference to the circulation of light meditation, which visualises the channels of the governor vessel and conception vessel.

Governor vessel 28: Yin crossing (yin jiao)
This point inside the mouth, between the upper teeth and the top lip, is the meeting of the governor vessel and the conception vessel, and in Daoist meditation techniques the placing of the tongue on the roof of the mouth is said to create a link between these yin and yang channels. Rubbing the point with the tongue stimulates the formation of saliva. Some Daoist practices advise the stimulation of saliva secretion during meditation as it is said to produce liquids full of essences, which when swallowed enrich the inner organs.

The linking of yin and yang at this level also relates to the two upper orifices – the mouth and the nose. The nose is said to be the gate of heaven, providing an entrance for the breath, the yang qi. The mouth is the door of the earth, receiving food and drink to create the yin essences of the body.

Illustrations tend to show the pathway of the governor vessel as a thin line following the spinal cord, running over the top of the head and penetrating the mouth, but the ancient presentations are always much more vague. They give the impression of a whole sphere of influence which extends over much of the back but also through the belly and up to the heart. Many of these pathway descriptions are symbolic and suggest the areas of influence of the yang, drawing particular relationships between the spine, as the channel for the most pure, heavenly energies, the heart, as the dwelling place of the spirits, and the brain. This meridian provides a link between the origin, the heart and the brain, the lower, middle and upper centres of transformation. Working on this channel with visualisation is central to many meditative practices. If the channel is blocked, the access to heaven is cut off; if it is open, light, subtle yang influences are able to penetrate – bringing life and strength to the lower abdomen, clarity and enlightenment to the brain; heavenly energies can flow downwards into the lower abdomen, bringing warmth and dynamism to this area of yin.

The conception vessel (ren mai)

From its beginning in the lower abdomen (shared with the du mai) and crossing in the area of the genitals, the ren mai or conception vessel flows up the centre front of the body (see Plate 5), creating a yin counterpart to the du mai. As the du mai brings movement, warmth, energy and clarity, the ren mai brings nutrition, humidity, darkness and protection.

The character ren, although generally translated in this context as conception, has the much wider meaning of to bear, to endure and to take the weight of something. The right part

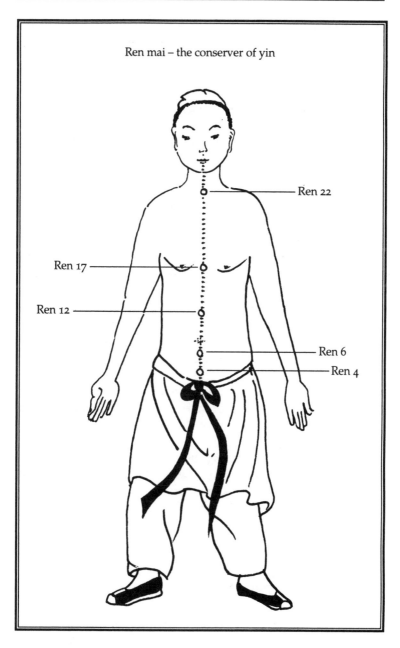

Ren mai – the conserver of yin

Ren 22

Ren 17

Ren 12

Ren 6

Ren 4

Plate 5

of the character literally represents the bamboo pole balanced across the shoulders and used to carry heavy objects that is still seen in many parts of the Far East. The left part of the character is the image of a human being. If this is exchanged for the image of a woman it means to bear a child.

So the conception vessel is responsible for the nourishment, the holding, the containing of a new life, but it is also responsible for the ability within each of us to renew and rebuild our own lives. It is responsible for the flesh and the blood and that earthly quality of breaking down and reabsorbing liquid and solid food to make it into a part of my own flesh and blood. But of course there can be no yin without yang and no life without an intermingling of these two qualities. Water without fire cannot create life, and the fire of the gate of life works within the water of the lower abdomen like the fire under the alchemist's crucible, allowing catalytic change.

The conception vessel is associated with yin and blood and form; the governor vessel with yang and qi and 'no-form'. The conception vessel needs this close link with the yang of the governor vessel, and its pathologies often relate to an excess of fluids, or an excess of matter in the form of lumps and masses, generally in the lower abdomen, suggesting an excess of yin and a lack of harmony between the yin and yang.

Conception vessel 1: Yin meeting (hui yin)
In some old texts this point, (between the anus and vagina in women, between the anus and scrotum in men), is given as the first point of the governor vessel, and the name yin meeting suggests the joining of the yang energy with the yin at this point. It has the function of anchoring the yang. It is mentioned in Daoist alchemical texts as a point of concentration in the exercises to retain and transmute seminal fluids and is also the starting-point for many important breathing exercises. A sense of tension in this area of the perineum is often a prerequisite for the performance of all kinds of breathing and movement exercises, both Indian and Far Eastern, suggesting that this rooting of the yang in the

depths of the body, the rooting of the yang within the yin, the spirit within the essence, is necessary for a good balance in the body.

This point is often treated with acupuncture for incontinence of the lower orifices; and exercise of the muscles in the perineum can have the same effect. The point can also be needled to anchor the yang when the patient has become disassociated or 'out of the body'.

Conception vessel 4: Gateway to the origin (guan yuan)
The three yin meridians in the legs (the liver, spleen and kidneys) meet and bind with the conception vessel at this point, on the front midline, roughly three inches above the pubic bone, bringing their yin nourishment from the earth. There is also a direct link with the governor vessel, and the name gateway to the origin suggests a mutual relationship with the gate of life. This is the yin centre of the lower abdomen, connected to the origin, and to all that is most precious, deep and intimate. It is the starting- and ending-point for much Oriental exercise and visualisation.

In Chinese medicine it is the major point for treating all yin deficiences and one of the main points used in acupuncture to treat infertility due to deficiency of yin or blood. It is often used with conception vessel 6, the sea of qi, to balance and strengthen both the blood and qi in the lower abdomen. In ancient texts it is often given as a point to use after great loss of blood during battle.

Conception vessel 6: Sea of qi (qi hai)
This point, one and a half inches below the navel, one and a half inches above conception vessel 4, symbolises the intermingling of yin and yang, the fire and water of the kidneys, bringing the fire of the gate of life to stimulate and invigorate the blood and liquids. The richness of the yin, essences and blood, need to be constantly warmed, moved and transformed by the yang. Below this point the energy of the conception vessel is very yin in quality. Here with the sea of qi there is an impulse of yang qi to enliven and invigorate the blood and essences – to prevent stagnation and accumulation. To keep a

balance between piling up and dispersing, solidifying and freeflowing.

Conception vessels 4 and 6 are important points to stimulate the lower energy centre and they are both frequently used in acupuncture and moxibustion treatment and as a focus for the attention in qi gong exercise and meditation. When working with them it is useful to remember the distinctions between them. Use the lower point when specifically working with the yin, the upper point when working more with the qi. In the lower abdomen both energies need to balance and intermingle, and a general concentration on the area of these two points is fine for general exercise.

Traditionally, in both qi gong and the meditation practices, women do not concentrate on the lower abdomen during menstruation, concentrating instead on the upper sea of qi between the breasts. The writings of women Daoists have suggested that the area of the chest may have been a preferred area of concentration for women generally, and that in fact the emphasis placed on the lower abdomen or hara has developed particularly within the Japanese Zen tradition.

Conception vessel 12: Central storehouse (zhong wan)
Halfway between the navel and the end of the sternum, this is the main treatment point for the stomach and the middle burner, the centre of the earth energy for the absorption and distribution of nourishment. As the points in the lower abdomen acted as a centre for the original energies, balancing original yin and original yang, this centre in the upper abdomen oversees the energy intake from food and drink and acts as a central point of distribution. And as the points in the lower abdomen relate to the kidneys and the functions attributed to the kidneys in Chinese medicine, so this centre relates to the spleen and stomach.

Conception vessel 17: Centre of the chest (tan zhong)
On the sternum midway between the two nipples, this point is also called the upper sea of qi. It is the centre responsible for all the rhythms and cycles within the body. These rhythms and cycles are controlled by the breath, and govern the

beating of the heart, the opening and closing of the pores of the skin and the smooth passage of food along the various gates and doors of the alimentary canal. The point is also the centre of the ancestral qi, which gathers all the qi together here, maintaining the body in the shape and form of its inherited pattern.

It is from this centre that the circulation of both qi and blood is controlled, and by controlling the breath we can in fact ultimately control those processes of the body that we usually assume to be automatic – like the beating of the heart and the workings of our digestive tract. If we can control our breath we can control our life. Life begins and ends with the breath, and whereas the centres in the lower abdomen were active during development in the womb, this centre is only truly active on the first intake of breath.

All Oriental exercise, massage and meditation requires awareness of the breathing, whether it is simply co-ordination of an outward movement with an outward breath, or the complex breath control of certain forms of Daoist yoga. The breath is primary. And whether the focus of concentration is on the lower abdomen or on the eyebrow centre, breathing always works to regulate the heart and lungs, to calm the spirit and still the mind. It is with this work on the breath that we gradually come to know and understand our bodies. The calmness and stillness that come from a quiet nervous system allow the body to speak its needs and begin to balance its disharmonies.

Conception vessel 22: Heavenly chimney (tian tu)

This point is in the hollow at the base of the neck. Around the neck are a group of points known as the windows of heaven. They provide access for the yin to the yang area of the head, allowing the richness of the essences and the cooling and humidifying effects of the yin to moisten the brain, the face and the upper orifices. The windows of heaven moisten the throat and the voice and allow clarity of speech, they bring moisture to the eyes, allowing clear vision, and to the ears and the nose. Each yin meridian tends to be associated with its particular orifice, for example, yin is brought by the liver to the eyes, by the lung to the nose, by the spleen to the mouth; they do so in fact by joining at these points with their associated yang meridians, allowing a complete interpenetration of the yang by the yin.

This particular point of the conception vessel, the sea of all the yin meridians, oversees the whole process and is responsible for the moistening and cooling of all the head and upper orifices. From the throat the ren mai flows into the mouth and joins with the du mai forming the primary circulation of yin and yang. An internal pathway flows upwards following the stomach meridian and enters the eye. By working with these two channels we aim to bring yin and yang into perfect balance and equilibrium, a state of stillness and calm, which is illustrated by the tai ji, the ying yang symbol. But in order for growth and development to be possible there must be dynamism, and within the extraordinary meridians this dynamism is brought by the penetrating vessel.

The penetrating vessel (chong mai)

After the dynamic balance of the first couple, the penetrating vessel, chong mai, is the third of the extraordinary meridians. As two is the number of balance and harmony, three is the number of movement and vitality, and the name chong means to rush, to surge and to penetrate. In terms of embryology, it is the activity of the chong mai that is said to form the limbs, as its energy bursts with the same kind of vitality as the liver from the original circle to surge into the legs. Its pathway is described as beginning with the same joint origin of the governor vessel and conception vessel, deep within the lower abdomen; it surfaces just above the pubic bone, either side of the conception vessel. From there it surges down into the legs following the pathway of the kidney meridian and penetrates into the earth at the sole of the foot (see Plate 6). An internal pathway rises and circles the mouth.

The penetrating vessel links the energies of the origin and of 'posterior heaven', associated with the kidneys, with those of 'anterior heaven', associated with the stomach, which

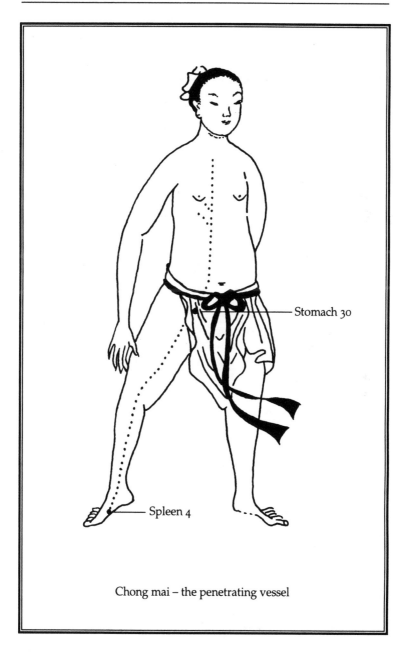

Stomach 30

Spleen 4

Chong mai – the penetrating vessel

Plate 6

means that it combines the inherited tendencies and constitutional energies with the ability to create usable energy from what we eat and drink.

The penetrating vessel has the ability to unite the power of yin and yang and to create a dynamic thrust of energy. It breaks out of the equilibrium of balance and harmony to create growth and change. Its various names in the classics stress that it can control yin and yang, blood and qi. Its pathway links the sea of qi in the abdomen, where it originates, with the sea of qi in the chest, where it disperses.

This meridian is often used in practice to provide movement where there is stagnation. It may be used to encourage the flow of a late period, or to help the yin energy to flow upwards and penetrate the chest, or it may be used to encourage the flow of energy into the legs in cases of weakness and immobility. Its action is dynamic, it penetrates and moves, balancing yin and yang, blood and qi.

Stomach 30: Surging qi (qi chong)

It is from this point, two inches either side of the midline at the level of the pubic bone, that the qi surges down into the legs and also up into the trunk, and in practice it is often used to harmonise the blood and the qi, and to help circulation both in the abdomen and in the legs.

Spleen 4: Yellow Emperor (gong sun)

This point, on the inside edge of the foot, just below the protruding bone, is called the master point for the penetrating vessel, and is used to activate the meridian. Amongst the extraordinary meridians only the conception vessel and governor vessel have their own points; the other extraordinary meridians share specific points with the 12 ordinary meridians. This point is used to invigorate the penetrating vessel and particularly to restore the balance between blood and qi. It also has a dynamic action that can break through stuckness and blockage. It is useful in many menstrual problems, particularly if there is obstruction to the flow.

The girdle vessel (dai mai)

As its name suggests, the dai mai, or girdle vessel, forms a belt around the waist and literally keeps the other meridians in their place. The term meridian implies a warp of threads on a weaving loom, all stretched at a particular tension to make the weaving of a pattern possible. All the meridians on the body follow this north–south axis, running from earth to heaven, heaven to earth; the girdle vessel is the only exception. Secured at the lower back at the level of the gate of life, the girdle vessel binds around the body, following the lower ribs to the side waist, and falling downwards to the level of the gate of origin (see Plate 7).

As with all belts, it is important that it has the correct tension. Too slack, and the meridians become loose and uncontrolled; too tight and there is constriction. Pathologies related to the girdle vessel often refer to the feeling of being seated in water up to the waist, or of the top of the body being unrelated to the bottom. In practice, women in particular tend to have problems with this meridian, often displaying a complete change in body shape below the waist. If the belt is too loose there may be excessive accumulation of liquids in the lower abdomen, which eventually dampen the fire of the gate of life.

An overtightening of dai mai may manifest as stiffness in the muscles, a lack of flexibility especially around the waist and lower back, but also emotionally in all kinds of rigidity of thought. Problems with the girdle vessel are also considered to be a major cause of vaginal discharges.

The main points associated with dai mai are Du 4 (gate of life), Ren 4 (gate to the origin) and also Gall-bladder 26.

Gall-bladder 26: Girdle vessel (dai mai)

Located at the side of the body at the level of the navel, this point is used to free the muscles, to regulate menstruation and to treat vaginal discharges. Its name is the same as that of the meridian, and it is the most effective point to treat general dai mai symptoms. Many of the side stretches mentioned in Parts 3, 4 and 5 activate this point and help the function of dai mai.

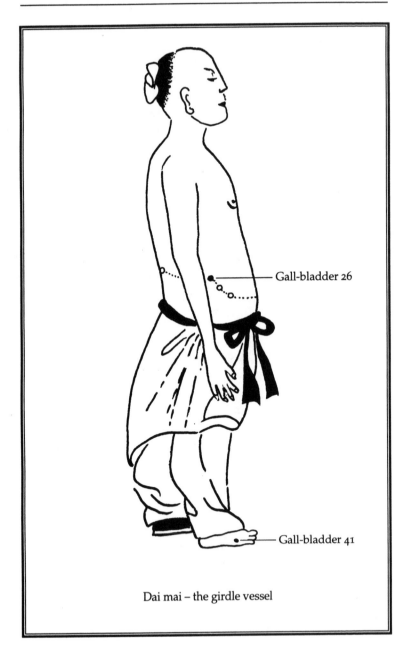

Gall-bladder 26

Gall-bladder 41

Dai mai – the girdle vessel

Plate 7

Gall-bladder 41: Overlooking tears (lin qi)
On the outer edge of the foot between the fourth and fifth toe joints, this point is the master point of the girdle vessel. It loosens the muscles and frees blockages around the waist and the ribcage, particularly in the area of the floating ribs. It is used in acupuncture to treat liver and gall-bladder qi stagnation. The meridians of the liver and gall-bladder run up the sides of the body, giving them the power to control movement and circulation at the sides of the body, but they can also be used to free all kinds of blockage and accumulation as the liver controls freeflow of any kind.

These four meridians form the basis from which the body shape can emerge. The governor vessel and conception vessel give the north–south axis and the primal balance of yin and yang; the penetrating vessel in the centre, combining yin and yang, blood and qi in a dynamic expression of life force; the girdle vessel creating volume and a balance between the top of the body and the bottom. The remaining four, two pairs of yin yang meridians, build on this first structure, giving rhythm and balance, and expanding into the limbs to give structure to the emerging system of the 12 ordinary meridians.

BALANCING AND INTEGRATING YIN AND YANG

Yin and yang qiao mai

We have seen that the first four of the extraordinary meridians all originate within the depths of the lower abdomen. Here with the qiao mai (usually translated as heel vessels) we move away from that central organisation with an upward flow of energy from the earth. The qiao mai begin together at the centre of the base of the heel and divide into yin and yang, the yin connecting with the inner ankle, the yang connecting with the outer ankle. This intimate relationship with the heel is reflected in the Chinese character 'qiao' which means to surge upwards, but also to stand in an upright and dynamic way, and is used in combination with other characters to describe agility. Classical commentators suggest that the qiao mai enable us to walk and run with agility. Heel in the Chinese also has a correspondence with the root, and these meridians are also said to provide our rooting in the earth.

The pathways differ in various texts, the older texts always more vague and symbolic, the later texts more precise. From their common beginnings in the centre of the heel, the yin qiao mai binds around the inner ankle and follows the inner leg to the area of the genitals. From there it rises and penetrates the throat, linking with chong mai, and upwards to the inner corner of the eye. The yang qiao mai rises from the heel, over the back, around the shoulders and into the throat. It rises to the inner corner of the eye, where it joins with the yin qiao, then doubles back and penetrates the back of the head (see Plate 8).

In many ways their pathways are an extension of the functions of the governor vessel and the conception vessel, enlarging and bringing precision to the yin yang balance. In the same way that the governor vessel and the conception vessel envelope the body, creating a circle around the head and trunk, the qiao mai extend this influence, creating a circle from their joint beginnings in the heel to their meeting at the eye, and are often referred to in Daoist exercise as 'the greater circle'. They are in charge of the balance between yin and yang, fire and water, blood and qi, nutrition and defence at all levels of the body, and particularly for attuning the body to the cycles of night and day. If your body is no longer functioning according to the natural rhythms and cycles of night and day, working with these meridians through exercise or massage of their master points can have great effect.

Kidney 6: Shining sea (zhao hai)

Below the inner ankle bone, this is the master point of yin qiao mai. It is on the kidney meridian and reflects the balance of water and fire. The kidneys are of the water element, but always indicate the balance of yin and yang, fire and water; in some of the old texts one kidney is related to yang and fire,

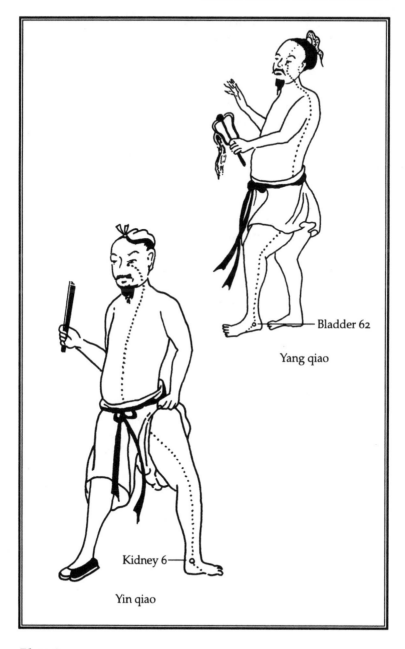

Bladder 62

Yang qiao

Kidney 6

Yin qiao

Plate 8

the other to yin and water. The character zhao, shining, is the image of the sunlight reflected on the water, and can be translated as shining or shimmering. The name suggests the power of the sun, the light, the fire on the water. The qiao mai create the unity between yin and yang, fire and water, top and bottom, night and day, and this point is particularly important to give the impetus for the yin to reach to upper parts of the body.

Traditionally it is often used to provide yin and moisture to the eyes and the throat and to treat insomnia.

Bladder 62: Extending meridian (shen mai)

Below the outer ankle bone, this is the master point of the yang qiao mai. Shen means to stretch and extend, but also to be at ease. From the heels the body is able to stretch upwards, to move forward. From their deep rooting within the earth, the qiao mai are able to give this agility of movement, and to circulate yin and yang qi from the heels to the top of the head.

Shen is also the character given to the ninth of the 12 earthly branches, relating to the time of day between three and five p.m. and to the optimum time for the bladder meridian. This is said to be the time when the yang welcomes the yin, as day turns to night, and suggests the ability of the qiao mai to be constantly moving between yin and yang, balancing and crossing each other and different levels of the body.

It is often used to treat headaches, and with Kidney 6 to balance sleeping patterns.

Yin and yang wei mai

The meaning of wei is to attach and anchor, to preserve and maintain. Both the qiao mai and the wei mai create balance and harmony between yin and yang in the body, but whereas the qiao mai begin together, have specific pathways and join again, creating one cycle of energy, the wei mai are quite distinct and separate. The yin wei looks after the yin, the yang wei looks after the yang. They do not meet or cross or interlink. In the early texts they are given no distinct pathways, the yin wei merely having the function of maintaining and anchoring the yin and governing the inside of the body, the yang wei of maintaining and anchoring the yang and governing the outside of the body.

From these basic functions we can elaborate that the yin wei is in charge of the blood and nutrition, the yang wei of the qi and defence. Where a channel is mentioned in later texts, the yin and yang wei have separate starting-points and their pathways do not cross. The yin wei is said to begin at the crossing of the yin (at point Kidney 9 on the calf), the yang at the meeting of all the yang (at point Bladder 63 on the outside of the foot; see Plate 9). Some later texts describe the yin wei as ending in the throat and merging with the ren mai, the yang wei ending at the back of the head and merging with the du mai.

The yang wei mai holds and contains all the yang meridians and all the yang functions of warming, moving, holding up and defending the exterior. The yin wei mai holds and contains all the yin meridians and all the yin functions of cooling, nourishing and protecting the interior. They are quite separate and distinct, not so much responsible for the balance between the yin and yang, as in the mutual exchange of the qiao mai, but responsible each for their own charge. Their functions are well illustrated by their master points.

Heart master 6: Inner gateway (nei guan)

On the internal face of the arm, about two inches above the wrist, the inner gateway, or passage to the interior, is located on the heart master or heart protector meridian (in modern books often called the pericardium), at the specific place where the meridian connects with the interior, and particularly with the heart. It is the main point in the body to free constriction in the chest and around the heart, and also builds the blood and the yin.

Triple heater 5: Outer gateway (wai guan)

On the external face of the arm, two inches above the wrist, and at the same level as the inner gateway, this point is used

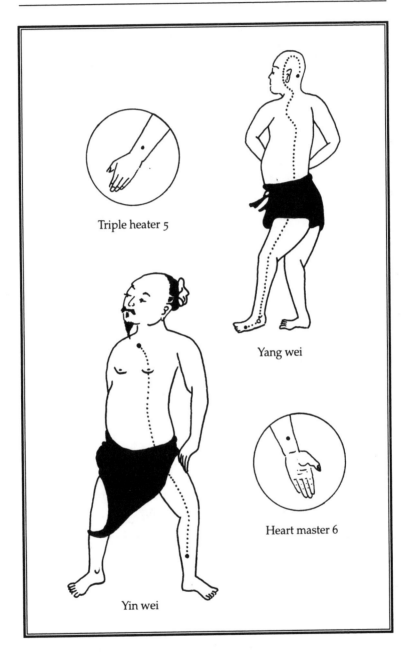

Triple heater 5

Yang wei

Yin wei

Heart master 6

Plate 9

to invigorate the circulation of qi, particularly in its ability to defend from external attack, for example by cold or wind. If there is plenty of qi circulating close to the surface of the body, the pores are able to open and close and the body is able to maintain its temperature. If this qi is weak, the body may be easily affected by the cold, which may cause an inner state of chills and fevers as the yin and yang are not properly balanced.

The muscles also operate at this external level, and the yang wei mai provides qi to the muscles. If this is deficient there may be muscle spasms and cramping or, in severe cases, weakness of the muscles to the extent that one can no longer grasp anything. The classical texts often say that if the yang wei is weak, one is unable to grasp anything with the hands, if the yin wei is weak, one is unable to grasp anything with the mind. These two points would be useful in treating both those conditions.

The du mai is master of the original yang, the ren mai protector of the original yin. The chong mai creates life through the conjunction of opposites, yin and yang, fire and water, blood and qi. The dai mai creates volume and space. Yin and yang qiao govern the rhythms and cycles of yin and yang, continually interpenetrating. They govern right and left, east and west, like the continual rising and setting of the sun. The yin wei mai binds and holds the yin and the blood; the yang wei mai binds and holds the yang and the qi. Together they create a network able to form the basis and foundation for the functioning of the 12 ordinary meridians with their complex interrelationships and associations to the five elements and the internal organs.

THE THREE CENTRES OF ENERGY TRANSFORMATION

Three centres of energetic interchange are referred to in Chinese medicine; they are located in the lower abdomen, the upper abdomen and the chest. They are usually called the three heaters or the three burning spaces, to suggest the alchemical processes of energy transformation that take place at these three levels.

In the centre of the chest, the upper burning space, the heart and lungs give a rhythm to the body and transform energy from the air we breathe. In the middle burning space, the stomach and spleen transform the food we eat into usable energy and are responsible for its distribution around the body. In the lower abdomen, or the lower burning space, our constitutional energies and inherited tendencies are stored, and the strength of this inherited energy, or original energy, determines the ability of the other two centres to perform their transformations, acting as a kind of catalyst in their alchemical processes. This energy of the lower burning space is related to the kidneys and determines fertility, development and growth.

When the practitioner of Oriental medicine takes the pulse in three positions on the wrist, it is the strength of these three energetic centres and their related organs that is being assessed. The lower heater contains the kidneys and bladder, and is also responsible for the functions of the intestines. The middle heater contains the digestive organs of the stomach and spleen, liver and gall-bladder, and the upper heater, the heart and lungs. Often the aim of treatment is to create balance and harmony between these three centres.

Many common problems can be seen as an imbalance between these three centres, and we often have strengths in one area and weaknesses in another. Emotional tendencies also play their part in this balance. Sexual and survival drives originate in the lower centre, the need for nourishment in the second centre, while the heart centre is the source of stillness and calm.

If the spleen energy is disturbed by overthinking or worry, there will be a knotting of the energy of the middle burning space, creating communication problems between the upper and lower centres. There may be agitation and insomnia, which are typical symptoms of the loss of harmony between fire and water affecting the heart and the spirit. On the other

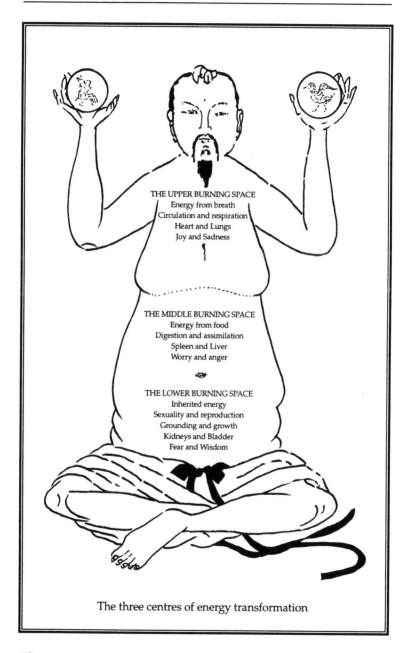

THE UPPER BURNING SPACE
Energy from breath
Circulation and respiration
Heart and Lungs
Joy and Sadness

THE MIDDLE BURNING SPACE
Energy from food
Digestion and assimilation
Spleen and Liver
Worry and anger

THE LOWER BURNING SPACE
Inherited energy
Sexuality and reproduction
Grounding and growth
Kidneys and Bladder
Fear and Wisdom

The three centres of energy transformation

Plate 10

hand, there may be loss of control over the lower orifices with nervous diarrhoea or the inability to hold urine.

THE LOWER BURNING SPACE

In simple five-element terms, this is the centre of water and of the kidneys, the root of our being and the root of our inherited energies. It is from the deep, dark, secret place that transformation is possible, as we saw with the image of the seed in winter, buried deep within the earth, the symbol of the potential for growth and transformation contained within the kidney energy. With their connection to the spinal cord and brain, and to the possibility of transforming fear into wisdom, the kidneys provide the basis for all possible change and evolution whether it is physical, emotional or spiritual.

But there are two important aspects of the lower energy centre, and as we have seen, in this area of the lower abdomen there is always a dynamic balance of water and fire, yin and yang. All three energetic centres are important for the transformation and transportation of fluids, and here in the lower burning space the main physical function is of separation of the pure and impure elements of food and drink, and the transformation of the less refined physical substances into energies that the body can use. The pure are reabsorbed into the body, the impure are excreted in urine and faeces. In *The Yellow Emperor's Classic* the lower heater is often compared to a drainage system carefully designed to channel water in the correct way. The small intestine absorbs nutrients and channels the solid waste into the large intestine and the liquids to be excreted to the bladder. Being the yang organ related to the fire element, the small intestine is the yang partner of the heart, and this ability to separate the pure and the impure, to make judgements and be discerning, is shared with the heart, which makes similar judgements in the realm of thoughts and emotions.

The large intestine is linked with the lungs and the metal element. Its function in the lower centre is to condense and finally to let go of that which is no longer appropriate for our physical growth and development.

It is the aspect of fire in the lower burning space that allows the recuperated liquids to be incorporated once more into the body. But it is not only liquids that are recuperated. During this whole process of digestion there is a constant breakdown of food into usable energy. The medical classics tell us that this final extraction of energy from food in the lower heater is transformed by the fire of the gate of life, the original fire, to create our defensive energy. This implies that if the fire aspect of the lower burning space is weak, there may be a lack of defence. Our immunity will be lowered, making us susceptible to colds and flus, viruses and bacteria or any other kind of external attack. In Japan in particular it is always considered to be of vital importance to keep the area of the kidneys warm and the fire of the lower heater strong. Without this fire in the lower heater there is no transformation and the body soon becomes listless and the will weak.

The lower heater is also the area of sexuality and fertility. And as we saw clearly with the joint pathways of the du mai and the ren mai, it is the constant intermingling of yin and yang, fire and water, blood and qi in this area that creates fertility. Most treatment for infertility aims to create the correct balance between the ability to create life and growth and the ability to nourish and hold.

In Chinese alchemy this lower energy centre is often pictured as a field being tilled by a simple ox-drawn plough, a symbolic representation of the repetitive work needed to transform the rough matter of the earth into a fertile field ready to provide growth and transformation. The action of the plough continually turning over the ground is replaced in alchemical practice with the repetitive action of the breath.

This lower centre of energetic transformation is stressed in much Eastern spiritual practice, particularly in Japan where concentration on the hara is common to most meditation and martial arts techniques. In the West, these lower centres are often neglected or considered dangerous, and practices will often stress concentration on the heart centre or on the centre between the eyebrows. The lower centre is the centre of our most powerful drives, those of survival and sexuality. If we attempt to cut off those drives as undesirable we risk losing our grounding and cutting our ties with the power of the earth. By bringing in consciousness and awareness we can begin to assist in our own evolutionary processes, gradually refining our energies so that we can live more effectively, more ecologically. Our kidneys are the root of our body-knowing. And in our attempts to raise ourselves up to a more spiritual way of being, we must be careful that we do not cut off from our instinctive feelings and our common sense.

The kidneys are the seat of our wisdom or know-how, literally enabling us to know how to live our lives. The ancient Chinese had no concept of the absent-minded profes-sor or the world-weary ascetic. Theirs is a practical wisdom which helps us to nourish the body and to regulate our energies as well as to live according to our destiny or mandate laid down by the blueprint of our ancestral energies. There is no division here between the physical and spiritual. As there can be no life without the interaction of heaven and earth, essence and spirit, the ancient Chinese did not attempt to nurture the spirit at the expense of the body. They saw the challenge of life on earth as the mutual co-existence of spirit and matter, the lower and the upper centres.

THE MIDDLE BURNING SPACE

The middle burning space is associated with the spleen and stomach and in the medical classics it is often called the sea of liquid and solid food. It is the function of the middle energy centre to take in food and break it down into some-thing that is so decomposed that it can be absorbed and used to maintain the body. If the middle burning space is strong it is able to take all that is useful in the food that we eat, and to assimilate it and make it our own with as little waste as possible. If it is not functioning well, even if our diet is sufficient, we may not be able to absorb what we need and much of value is lost. This is the reason why Oriental practitioners tend to assess the function of the spleen and stomach before suggesting changes in diet or even dietary supplements, for very often it is not our diet that is lacking but our ability to absorb and transform.

There are many stories of Daoist adepts able to exist on a few grains of rice, and these stories are no doubt based on the idea that their ability to create energy from food is so advanced that they waste nothing. They expend less energy because they 'follow the way' which often means the path of least resistance. If you do not meet resistance, you use less energy. Our modern lifestyles mean that we often eat on the run, have meetings over lunch and don't give our food much attention. Some of us can cope with this without seriously affecting our health. But if our earth element is weak, if our stomach and spleen are unable to transform and transport as well as they should, we may need to focus more on our eating habits. We will look at this again in Part 4. The process of reclaiming the wisdom of the body is to do with making unconscious or semi-conscious acts fully conscious. It concerns acting with awareness. Eating three grains of rice with full consciousness, chewing them carefully and extracting every element of nutrition may be just as nourishing as grabbing a sandwich as we rush from one meeting to another.

The spleen and stomach work together as a yin/yang couple, with the stomach receiving and processing the food and sending the purest essences to the spleen. The spleen is said to separate these essences into the five tastes and to send them to their appropriate organs: the sour taste to the liver, the bitter taste to the heart, the pungent taste to the lungs, the salty taste to the kidneys, while the sweet taste remains in the spleen. The five tastes are an important part of the concept of resonance within the five elements, and much of Chinese dietary theory is based on them. Each organ thrives on its own associated taste, but can also be damaged by an excess. A small amount of the salty taste strengthens the kidneys, but an excess will weaken them. A herb with a sour taste may be included within a herbal formula as it is said to 'enter the liver'. This herb will then be called the messenger herb, as it directs the herbal formula to the appropriate part of the body. Only the purest of the essences of food are able to pass through the filtering system of the diaphragm into the upper burning space where they are able to complete the formation of blood.

In the realm of thoughts, ideas and impressions, it is the spleen and its energetic centre that takes in information from the outside world, processes it and, according to the Chinese classics, presents it to the heart. If the spleen is weak it can be inundated by impressions and by other people's ideas and find it difficult to distinguish the useful from the useless.

Over the past 25 years, Dr Hiroshi Motoyama has performed a series of tests on psychics and healers in his research institute in Tokyo, with his device for measuring the function of the acupuncture meridians. The research found that those who were tested fell into two significant groups – those who could receive and those who could transmit. The receivers – individuals who displayed what would usually be called extra-sensory perception and could receive an image in their mind transmitted by another – often exhibited irregularity in their spleen meridian function. For example, the meridian would be very erratic, swinging from a vastly increased to a vastly diminished energy.

The transmitters – including many healers – tended to show irregularity in the heart and heart master meridians. A third group was discovered who showed abnormalities in the kidney and bladder meridians, related to the lower energy centres. It is fascinating that this group tended to have strong psychic abilities which were not yet under their conscious control but were exhibited spontaneously. The Indian tradition reminds us that concentration on the centres in the lower abdomen may promote psychic phenomena, but that these should be ignored until they can be controlled by the intelligence of the heart.

When I accompanied Dr Motoyama to the Philippines in the late seventies as a part of his ongoing study of the phenomenon of psychic surgery, we tested many of the healers and also those receiving healing. The patients were tested both before and ten minutes after healing, and irrespective of the site of their 'surgery', all patients displayed an increase in the energy of the spleen meridian after healing. In some people it would be minimal, in others very exaggerated, but the pattern was clear, suggesting that healing energy of this kind is received in the body via the spleen meridian.

So the spleen centre is the place where energy and information can enter the body and psyche and, as with all points of entry and exit in Chinese medicine, it must be guarded. It is good to be open to outside influence, but not too open. In Japan possession by ghosts and by other people's ideas is rooted in a long tradition and taken very seriously. We attract by our neediness and our desire, and in the same way that our taste should be able to distinguish what is good or bad for our bodies so our purpose is able to guard us from the invasion of unsuitable ideas and influences.

THE UPPER BURNING SPACE

In Chinese medicine the heart is the centre of human life. In Confucian terms, it was the emperor of the other organs, capable of wise, discerning judgement. The Daoist texts portray the heart as the dwelling-place of the spirits or influences from heaven. The heart/mind must be quiet to attract the spirits, and the preparation of the heart is likened to the preparation of a nest for a bird – if the proper home is found, the birds will stay; if there is agitation, the birds will fly away. The spirits represent the presence of heaven within us; they are attracted by an empty peaceful heart, but they do not remain in the heart alone. Through the blood and the circulation of the blood they take this spiritual influence down to the very cells of the body.

All circulation of qi and blood takes place from the upper burning space. It is the rhythm of the breath and the rhythm of the heart that create this ability to circulate and it is the presence of the spirits of the heart that is said by the ancient Chinese to give blood both its red colour and its intelligence. The Chinese have maintained for over 2,000 years that the blood has consciousness, and this is being borne out by recent discoveries in biophysics of the neuropeptides, intelligent hormone-like substances that circulate in the bloodstream.

The spirit/intelligence is present throughout the whole body via the network of meridians and via the blood, the circulation of which is governed by the heart and lungs in the upper heater.

This centre in the chest is also the centre for the so-called 'ancestral energy'. With the original energy (yuan qi) and the original essence (jing), the ancestral energy (zong qi) is the third of the inherited or pre-natal energies. As the yuan qi connects with the origins of life and enables energetic transformations within the body, and the jing forms the material basis for life and development, the zong qi is said to give the individual stamp to the being. It is called ancestral energy because it is concerned with the individual lineage, the inherited traits and tendencies, but the Chinese character 'zong' also has the meaning of a gathering, and it is the gathering of energies here in the area of the heart that gives individual expression to the being: the mark of individuality or personality given by the presence of the spirits.

Modern commentators suggest that the ancestral energy is linked with immunity, in that it is able to recognise that which is mine and of my own type, and differentiate and exclude that which is foreign to me. The defensive qi, which also plays its part in immunity, is formed in the lower burning space by the action of the fire of the gate of life and is distributed from the upper sea of qi. We saw with the movement of the extraordinary meridian, the chong mai, that part of its function was to join these two energetic centres, linking the centre of fire in the lower abdomen with the centre of fire in the chest. Many Daoist breathing exercises aim to establish a good communication between these two vital centres.

The triple burner meridian belongs to the fire element and, along with its yin partner the heart master, governs what is called ministerial fire, linking the energetic centres of transformation. The heart is the emperor fire, and controls all that is of the nature of heaven and the spirit. The triple burner and heart master govern the more practical aspect of fire, creating movement and heat, transforming and moving body fluids and blood. At this upper centre, all the qi gathers to be distributed around the body by the blood vessels under the control of the heart and by the acupuncture meridians, which begin their circulation in the lungs.

The lungs are often called the 'heavenly canopy', their upper lobes forming the highest extension of the internal organs. In the upper burning space this heavenly canopy acts to attract all rising vapours and qi and to direct them downwards. The balance between the kidneys, which root the qi, and the lungs, which have this action of controlling the upper extension of qi and vapours, works to ensure that the lungs are not blocked and congested. Congestion in the lungs may cause breathing problems and asthma, and the Oriental practitioner would need to differentiate between asthma relating to a deterioration of the lung function and asthma relating to a deterioration of the kidney function. Accompanying signs and symptoms would enable the practitioner to make a differential diagnosis, as we will see in Part 5. The lungs also diffuse the liquids and moisten the skin, and it is the understanding of this connection which makes Chinese medicine so effective in treating related lung and skin problems, such as asthma and eczema.

Whereas the work in the lower centre involved the transmutation of energies of a physical nature, ensuring the health and vitality of the upper centre often involves the control and transformation of emotional energies. A peaceful heart is a heart unruffled by emotions; it is not a heart that does not feel emotion but a heart that feels with intensity while remaining unmoved from its own centre. The emotions are energetic movements and the Daoist sages likened them to the wind blowing through the reeds, and the wind in the willow tree, which is able to move and bend but always remains rooted and strong, its very pliability providing its greatest strength.

The interdependence of the fire and water, the heart and the kidneys, can be seen again here – the kidneys providing the stability and rooting which enables the heart to be light and pliable and empty. All qi gong, tai ji and martial arts have this as their underlying principle. The lower body is strong and firm, the two legs providing a rooting into the ground of the dynamic hara energy. Above the waist there is lightness, flexibility, the feeling of floating upwards as the body expands, suspended between heaven and earth.

The appreciation of the need to be able to 'sit quietly' permeates all Eastern culture. Particularly in China and Japan where yin yang theory forms the basis of all cultural life, it is always apparent that activity must be followed by stillness, physical activity by physical stillness, mental activity by mental stillness.

Many meditation techniques aim to still the mind by concentration on the breath, concentration on an object or, as in tai ji, for example, concentration on the movement of the body.

The early Daoist sages stressed stillness, shutting down the senses until no impressions are presented to the mind, no seeing, no hearing, remaining quietly within. But having shut down the communication with the outside world one is faced with the turmoil of the inner world of thoughts and feelings. The early Daoist writings liken the mind/heart to a pool of water agitated by the wind. Regular breathing and focusing the mind allow the pool to become calm again – a clear surface that reflects reality with the precision of a mirror. A mind disturbed by emotion cannot reflect reality.

But what creates the movement of the wind? What creates the over-activity of the emotions? According to the early Daoist writings it is desire. Desire keeps the mind active. Meng zi, one of the early Confucian writers, said that 'For nourishing the spirit, nothing is better than emptying it of desires'. Zhuang zi, a Daoist contemporary of Meng zi, states that the mind of the sage is not still simply because he thinks it should be still – the mind of the sage is still because 10,000 things are not enough to disturb his stillness.

The idea is to be empty without struggling to be empty. To be calm without struggling to be calm. Just let go. Just breathe. Just be.

PART 3

BALANCING HEAVEN AND EARTH

General Exercises

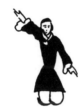

Approaching this part of the book, I cannot help but feel cautious; cautious of advising more exercise, more ideas on diet, more things to think about and be confused by; more pressure to make us feel guilty that we are not doing enough. In a busy city-centre practice I often advise patients to 'not do'. To take time out. To rest more. And also within their 'doing' to try to achieve a sense of relaxation. So although the purpose of this section is to introduce exercises, self-massage and other ways to use the philosophy of Chinese medicine to shed light on specific imbalances, the aim is also to keep it simple. Don't expect to do everything. Pick and choose the things that appeal and those that seem relevant. The exercise is not strenuous; it is more about relaxation and concentration than bending and stretching. Qi gong is designed to follow the body's natural energy flow: the more you relax and release, the more you feel that the movement is happening naturally, of its own accord. You literally do nothing but follow.

'Sitting still, doing nothing' was an activity favoured by the ancient Daoists. They sat because they felt at one with heaven and earth. There was no reason to move, just to be. Nowadays we are trying to bring that sense of oneness into everyday life, not to become a recluse on a mountaintop or a nun in a nunnery, but just to live. So within our daily lives, within our roles of working, parenting, socialising – being normal human beings – we need to find some space for stillness, to experience life's ups and downs, traumas and crises, but to do so with lightness. We need to listen to the lessons of the four seasons and understand the patterns of change and transformation, letting go of the old to make way for the new. And we need not expect perfection but learn to be a bit easier on ourselves. Humanity is in the process of becoming and our growth comes through trial and error. Better to try and err than to avoid trying through fear of failure.

ORIENTAL EXERCISE

In all therapeutic exercise there must be three components – movement, breath and concentration of intent. Chinese exercise begins with movement, but when the correct breathing and concentration is achieved there may be no more need of the external action; the breath and the intent have the most power. A simple exercise such as stretching the fingers may be performed casually, giving stretch and stimulation to the muscles and blood circulation, or it may involve concentration and intent, activating the qi or life force. In stretching out your fingers you can imagine the flow of qi in the meridians through the arms into each fingertip and projecting as far as the horizon; or you can sit while watching television stretching and clenching the fists. Both have their usefulness; it just depends what you are trying to achieve. To give the hands more suppleness all movement is good. To activate deep levels of self-healing and self-awareness, concentration is everything.

Some of the movements are generally balancing and can be of benefit to everyone; others are more specific and require some information from Parts 1 and 2 to apply effectively. If in doubt keep it simple. After 25 years of yoga, tai ji and qi gong practice, I have come back to the most simple teachings, and to the belief that it is not so much what you do but the way you do it that is important. When I first studied tai ji in the Far East, the group was young and forever looking for new styles and techniques. I practised with swords and envied those who had mastered complex animal forms. It was fun. Then I came across a qi gong teacher, a Zen monk who had travelled to India and spent much of his time wandering with his rice bowl. We studied with him when we could and learnt something very different. We learnt to stand still. I finally realised that it was much more difficult to achieve stillness than outward form.

It is easy to think that we are doing nothing if there is not a lot of movement involved. But it is the constant repetition of the same action, whether of the body or the breath, that can finally break down the old destructive pattern and create a new, more beneficial one, like the symbolic ploughing of the field in Daoist meditation. We are literally creating new energetic patterns that allow the body to function more effectively. Old tendencies and habits keep the body/mind from moving forward, keeping it trapped in old patterns of disharmony that prevent natural healing.

Since those early days I have experienced qi gong and other forms of Oriental exercise in many forms with many teachers, each adding something to the complete pattern. But only recently have I experienced the joy and expansion that comes with a practice that is rooted in the energies of heaven and earth and in my understanding of the bodily landscape. With Chinese exercise as well as medicine, it is easy to carry out the motions but to forget the root, to perform the actions but without understanding why. If we can begin to feel ourselves to be part of the earth, drawing energy and nourishment from the earth through the yin meridians in our feet, and part of heaven, drawing energy down through our head and our hands, warming and invigorating, clarifying and enlightening, we can begin to tune in to the universal energies. My hope is that this practice will not be a chore but something that can become part of our lives and a source of joy.

We may find that we have a constitutional type, either active or passive, yin or yang, hot or cold, and can create our main focus around that particular imbalance, adding variations depending on circumstances and energy cycles. Chinese medicine emphasises the treatment of the individual in the now, and our needs are constantly changing. If our current problems are insomnia and palpitations, we need stillness and quiet to calm the heart and settle the spirit. If we have irritation or anger we need vigorous movement to rebalance the flow of energy in the liver meridian. If we have headaches from overthinking, we can breathe into the lower abdomen, or massage the feet. If we are drowsy and sluggish, we can massage the head and exercise the neck.

The important thing is to be aware, constantly asking, 'How does this make me feel?' Unused muscles ache when they become active again, but it is a good ache that sometimes needs to be worked through, relaxed into, released. A sharp stabbing pain in the knee while you are trying to sit between your heels is not good, and it needs attention – change your position, use a higher cushion, but don't ignore it. If you are working with exercises to open your chest and strengthen your lungs, it is natural to experience some aches and pains in the shoulders and upper back. These tight muscles need to be loosened and given space. But be gentle. Don't punish yourself. Feel as if you are massaging the muscles with your movement, not forcing them to stretch. Ten minutes a day is much more effective than working hard for an hour then forgetting for a week. Never force, remember to breathe and most important – relax.

LIFESTYLE

In the clinic, those patients who tend to make little progress are often those who are unable to make any changes to their lifestyle. That is always a matter of individual choice. But until we can see that our lifestyles and habitual patterns are often the cause of our illnesses, we can do little to heal ourselves. We may make temporary progress, but the patterns of disharmony tend to recur.

Our bodies, minds and spirits often suffer because we are afraid of change, afraid to move forward and let go. We become addicted to our present circumstances, to our pleasures, to our pains, to our belongings, to our lifestyles. And often we are addicted to the idea that to progress is to have more. So we get caught in an upward spiral of activity, which often wears us out, or in a downward spiral of depression because our desires are unfulfilled. But would we be willing to accept a lower standing of living in order to free up our time and make less demand on our energy? Would we be willing to make do with less so that we could spend more time with our children? Would we be willing for our children to have less so that we could live less stressful and more meaningful lives with them?

So-called New Age teachings have much to say about fulfilling our potential, but that does not necessarily mean more money, more fame, more cars and more real estate. Ecology tells us that we must begin to think down; think conservation; think equality; think sharing. The patterns of the seasons teach us in the most simple way that expansion must be followed by contraction, gaining by letting go. If that basic law of nature is not followed, if there is expansion, and more expansion and more expansion, there will eventually be catastrophic contraction causing great chaos and loss of life. It is the same with our bodies. If we work and work and push and push, and take pills to keep our bodies going because we have no time to rest, we invite a catastrophic collapse. Nature will take its course and we can choose to work with it or to work against it.

We may stay in situations where we feel secure, but our energies are stagnating. Our society, stressing insurance and investment, security and protection against any possible unforeseen circumstance, creates fear of change. We protect ourselves to the point where we no longer experience life, insuring ourselves against life itself.

Appropriate lifestyle is a completely individual thing. Some people have good energy and thrive on hard work. Some would be much healthier if they worked harder. Some of us stagnate, while others burn out. To find out what is best for us may take time, time to tune in to our bodies, our cycles, our needs. Sometimes our minds tell us one thing and our bodies another, but in fact, most of us know. Learn to accept your body as your teacher. Learn to listen to your body as well as your head; trust your feelings and begin to reclaim your body's wisdom.

BASIC QI GONG POSE

The most basic qi gong movements are designed to balance the energies of heaven and earth by following the natural flow of the yin and yang meridians in the body. This primary balancing exercise can be done by anyone at any time. Using the imagination and concentration, it can become a powerful tool for rebalancing and replenishing the body's energy.

Standing with the feet parallel and shoulder-width apart, slightly bend the knees. The feet should feel in contact with the ground, so spend a few moments checking that the balance is equal between the heels and the toes, the outer and inner edge of the foot. In the centre of the sole of the foot, the kidney meridian flows into the ground, giving rooting and stability to the body. Begin to imagine these roots growing through the feet down towards the centre of the earth.

The lower part of the body should feel solid and strong, completely balanced. Allow the body to sway backwards and forwards and from side to side to get the feel of your feet planted firmly on the ground.

Bringing your attention to the hips, put your hands on your hip bones and check that the left and right hips feel the same height. Rotate the hips a little while, keeping the feet solidly anchored to the ground. Consciously tilt the pelvis forward, stretching the lower part of the spine and slightly contracting the lower abdomen. This is a feeling or sensation more than a real muscular contraction, and don't worry if you can't quite feel it. It will come.

Close your eyes and just concentrate on your weight and gravity. The whole area below the waist should feel heavy and solid. Imagine your weight sinking down, through the waist, through the hips, down through the legs into the feet and through the soles of the feet deep into the earth. Feel rooted as a tree feels rooted.

THE MOVEMENTS

1. Let the hands rest gently on the lower abdomen wherever they feel comfortable. Bring your attention to your breath, breathing naturally and regularly (Fig. 1).

2. When the body feels completely relaxed, take a breath in, drawing the hands slowly apart, and at a distance of two or three inches from the body follow the line of the central energy channels (ren mai, Plate 5, and chong mai, Plate 6) from the lower abdomen to the chest (Fig. 2).

3. With the hands in front of the chest and the elbows raised, begin to exhale, move the hands across the chest, fingers pointing inwards towards the armpits, and gradually, with the exhalation, stretch the arms to a fully extended horizontal position, following the yin meridians flowing from the chest, along the internal face of the arm into the fingertips (Fig. 3).

4. Take a few deep breaths and with another inhalation stretch the arms and hands out and move them upwards as if embracing the heavens. Breathe out with the hands stretched above the head (Fig. 4).

5. After a few breaths, slowly bring the hands down to just above the top of the head, and down over the back of the head and neck to the shoulders, tracing the surface of the body but keeping the hands a few inches away (Fig. 5).

6. Bring the hands slowly to the front of the body, with the fingers and the concentration still pointing inwards to the spine. The breathing is natural (Fig. 6).

7. The hands follow the centre front and around the lower ribcage, while the concentration remains on the spine. The hands finally come to rest on the back at waist level, over the kidneys. Take a few breaths (Fig. 7).

8. On an exhalation, bend forward, follow the yang meridians on the back of the legs with the hands, until the hands reach the floor. Bend the knees as much as is necessary. Remain for a few moments contacting the yin and the earth (Fig. 8).

9. With the hands now on the inside, yin part of the legs draw the yin energy up through the legs into the groin and come to rest on the lower abdomen (Fig. 9).

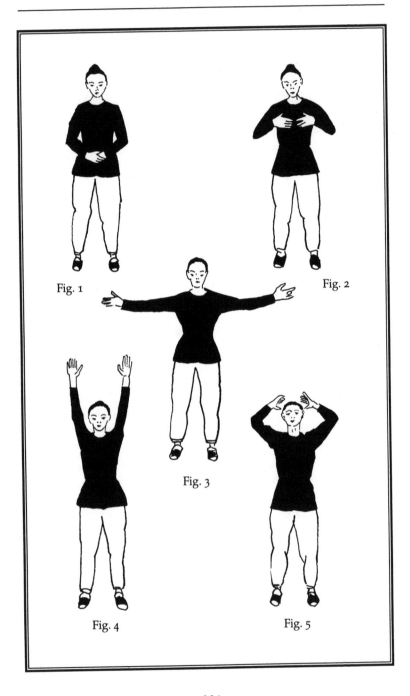

Fig. 1

Fig. 2

Fig. 3

Fig. 4

Fig. 5

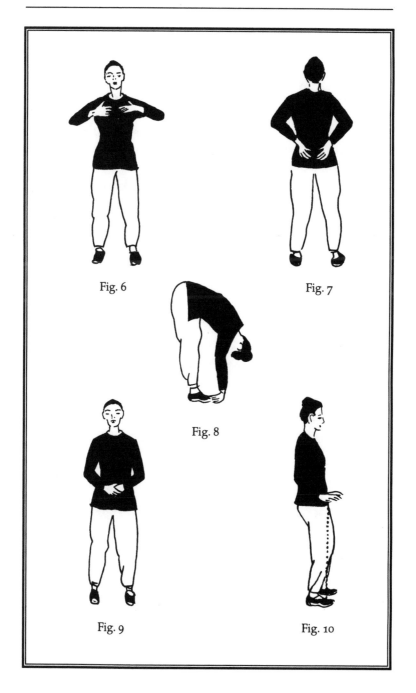

Fig. 6

Fig. 7

Fig. 8

Fig. 9

Fig. 10

This forms one cycle and should be repeated many times until the movements become fluid. They can be done very slowly, pausing for a few minutes at the major points, or very quickly, as if sweeping the meridians with the hands, using one in-breath up from the feet until the hands are above the head, and one out-breath to continue the cycle back down to the feet. This simple set of movements can be used in many ways and with subtle variations in many different situations and forms the basis for all qi gong movement.

FOCUSING THE ATTENTION

As you become more familiar with the movements, pay attention to each area. Remembering the function of each part of the body as you move through the positions helps to focus the concentration.

The lower abdomen:
Beginning in the lower abdomen, we imagine the primal beginnings of life with the three extraordinary meridians, the du mai, ren mai and chong mai, having their joint origin here. The acupuncture points gate to the origin and sea of qi are covered by the hands in the starting position. At the end of any exercise, the hands return to this position, centering and returning everything to the source. The three yin meridians of the legs, the kidney, spleen and liver meridians, all meet in the lower abdomen (Fig. 1).

The centre of the chest:
The ren mai and chong mai rise up the centre of the body, and the chong mai, along with the three leg yin meridians, disperse into the chest. This action is followed by the hands, pausing over the point, the central palace, in the centre of the chest. This is the centre of all circulation, all rhythms and regulations, the centre of the heart and lungs. And it is the heart and lung meridians that flow from the chest into the inner arms and through the palm of the hand to the fingertips (Fig. 2).

The centre of the palm:
The acupuncture point in the centre of the palm of the hand is connected with the heart. It is the fire point of a fire meridian and as such is a very powerful expression of yang. It is through these heart points at the centre of the palm that much hand healing is said to take place. It is the place where energy is most easily emitted. As you perform the hand movements of the basic qi gong exercises, concentration may be on the centre of the palm and many people begin to feel a tingling sensation there while performing the exercises. This is quite normal. Some people prefer to imagine the energy moving through the fingertips, others through the palm. In certain positions, one may feel more natural than the other. Just play with it. See which feels right for you (Fig. 3).

The top of the head:
As you bring your hands down over the top of your head you may begin to feel sensitivity at the crown of the head. This is the acupuncture point bai hui, one hundred meetings, on the governor vessel, corresponding with the position of the crown chakra. This is a great accumulation of the yang energy from heaven at the top of the head, which penetrates the brain and runs down the back of the head to the shoulders (Figs 4–5).

The back of the neck:
At the level of the shoulders all the yang meridians meet and circulate, forming a circle of energy around the shoulders and collar-bone. The acupuncture point da zhui, great hammer, where the bone protrudes at the top of the back, is an important point to regulate all the yang meridians in this area. It is on this point that we focus attention as we bring the hands down to the back of the shoulders (Fig. 5).

The kidneys:
The hands trace the front ribcage as the concentration remains on the spine, until they meet at the back of the waist over the kidneys. This is the gate of life, the point on the du mai at the

level of the kidneys and the origin. As the hands get warmer throughout the exercise, we can rest them over this point to stimulate the kidney energy and the general yang function in the lower parts of the body (Fig. 7).

The soles of the feet:
The hands move down the back of the legs bringing the yang all the way down to the feet, aiding circulation and warming the feet and legs. The acupuncture point in the centre of the sole of the foot is yong quan, gushing spring, the first point of the kidney meridian, bringing moisture and nourishment from the earth via the yin. This is the only meridian which does not begin or end at the tips of the fingers or toes, and possibly symbolises the great affinity of the kidneys and water with the primal yin energies drawn directly from the earth (Fig. 8).

The yin meridians from the feet flow up the inner part of the legs, the liver meridian encircling the genitals before all meeting together with the conception vessel (ren mai) in the lower abdomen (Fig. 9).

Balancing the five elements and the five directions:
This basic qi gong exercise expresses the cycle of the elements, the directions and the seasons. From the centre (Fig. 1) moving outwards with the horizontal expansion of the wood element and spring (Fig. 3); stretching upwards with the fire element and summer (Fig. 4); closing in again and returning to the centre for the contraction of metal and autumn (Figs 5 and 6), and moving downwards, contacting the earth and the depths for water and winter (Figs 7 and 8).

SIMPLIFIED MOVEMENTS

1. The same effect can be gained by using a simplified movement, beginning in the same way, but as the hands come down the front of the body, instead of going around the back to the kidneys, just gently push down with the hands until they are level with the lower abdomen and facing down-

wards. Imagine the centre of the palm aligned with the centre of the foot, and pushing down into the centre of the earth. After a few moments raise the hands again for a new cycle (Fig 10).

2. Sitting:
Another version may be performed in the sitting position: beginning with the hands over the lower abdomen, slowly stretch the arms outwards in the horizontal expanding movement; stretch upwards, then slowly bring the arms down to the shoulders, pushing downwards at the front of the body and resting the hands gently on the abdomen.

EXERCISES TO STIMULATE THE FLOW OF QI IN THE MERIDIANS

These exercises are commonly practised in both China and India. In yoga practice they are called pawanmuktanasana, or dispelling the wind postures. Both Indian and Chinese medical theory explain wind as a perverse energy that can lodge within the joints of the body. It causes stiffness and arthritis and can lead to serious internal problems if not addressed. Dr Hiroshi Motoyama learnt this particular set of exercises from Swami Satyananda of the Bihar School of Yoga, and adapted them according to his understanding of the acupuncture meridians. When practised with an appreciation of the flow of the acupuncture meridians, these exercises become a dynamic alternative workout.

During the time I spent in Tokyo they were taught to many of the elderly members of the Tamamitsu shrine with extraordinary results. Again they are very simple, but it is the regularity of practice and focus of attention that makes them so effective. They are usually performed sitting on the floor, but can even be adapted to be used lying in bed. If you can move little else, stretching the fingers and toes, the wrists and ankles provides essential stimulation to the acupuncture meridians. All meridians have their terminal points at the tips of the fingers and toes, and source points around the wrists and ankles. Stimulation to the extremities ensures that the energy does not stagnate even if we are unable to get out of bed.

A quicker standing version is given at the end of the section. This more vigorous routine is performed in various ways as a warm-up for all East Asian martial arts.

Moving through the body from the toes to the hips, the fingers to the shoulders, and finally to the head and neck, these exercises stimulate the joints, the muscles and tendons, the circulatory system and the meridian system at all major points of stagnation throughout the body. As we work through the body, we will also introduce a few simple self-massage techniques to enhance the effect. Some movements are performed with attention to the breath, others not. But at all times the breathing is regular and the concentration is maintained on the area you are working on.

METHOD

Sitting with the legs stretched out in front, with the hands supporting the weight of the body beside the buttocks, feel that the buttocks are even on the floor. Concentrate on the breath, breathing in and out a few times until a natural rhythm is achieved.

Toes:
1. With an inhalation curl the toes in, exhale and push the toes away and apart. Repeat ten times. Imagine as you breathe that the qi energy in the meridians is projected through the tips of the toes. This stimulates the well points at the tips of the toes, the beginning and ending points of the acupuncture meridians (Fig. 11).

The meridians in the feet are the bladder meridian at the outside of the heel, running down to the outside of the little toe. The gall-bladder meridian is just inside the bladder meridian, running over the front of the foot to end in the fourth toe. The stomach meridian runs down the centre front of the foot, terminating in the second toe. These are the three yang meridians of the foot, and they run down the body from the head.

The three yin meridians begin in the feet and flow upwards to disperse into the chest. The liver meridian runs next to the stomach, and ends in the inside of the big toe. The spleen meridian flows along the side of the foot and into the outside of the big toe. The kidney meridian binds around the inner ankle-bone and descends to the bottom of the foot. It is the only meridian with its first point not on the fingers and toes.

While stretching the toes we may notice that some move more easily than others and this may suggest a weakness in that particular meridian. Even if the toes themselves do not move easily, use the imagination to push the qi through the tips of the toes and with practice they will become more responsive. Walking with bare feet or exercise sandals will help feet that have been too restricted.

If the big toe is bent towards the foot and you have difficulty moving it outwards, this may suggest a weakness of the spleen, or possibly that the wood energy of the liver is overpowering the earth energy of the spleen. Concentrate on the big toe and try to move it outwards. Again, even if the toe does not physically move, the energy will begin to move, and this is a useful way to strengthen the spleen meridian. The first three points of the spleen meridian, all on the outside of the big toe, have a very powerful effect, and concentration and movement here is very beneficial.

Ankles:
2. With the legs stretched and the heels on the floor, breathe in and pull the feet towards the body, breathe out and stretch the feet away. Repeat ten times (Fig. 12). Keeping the legs quite still and the heels on the floor, rotate the right ankle clockwise five times, anti-clockwise five times. Repeat with the left, moving slowly and paying attention to any stiffness or pain. By becoming aware of imbalances, these exercises can become as much a means of diagnosis as of treatment, helping you decide which particular meridians may need special attention (Fig. 13).

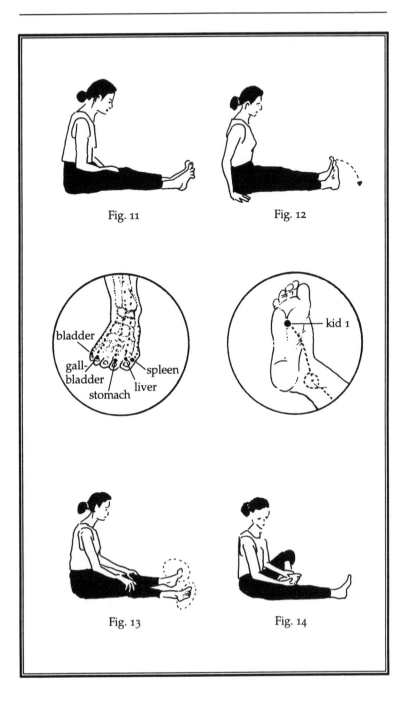

Fig. 11

Fig. 12

bladder

gall-
bladder

stomach

spleen

liver

kid 1

Fig. 13

Fig. 14

Foot massage:

3. Holding the right foot in both hands, rest it on the left leg. Massage the sole of the foot with the thumbs, paying attention to the area around Kidney 1 (gushing spring). This may be sensitive, and the thumbs should be used in stroking rather than prodding movements. Allow the two thumbs to come together at the centre of the foot, and massage outwards. You will know what feels good.

With the thumb and forefinger lightly pinch along the outside edge of the foot to stimulate the bladder meridian. Massage and pull the little toe. Pull each of the toes in turn. If you noticed earlier any toes which seemed particularly immobile, give them an extra massage and an extra pull. Repeat with the left foot (Fig. 14).

Stretch the legs out in front of you and shake them, with the heels and buttocks still in contact with the floor.

Knees:

4. Holding the right leg under the thigh take a breath in. As you breathe out stretch the foot away and straighten the knee. Point the toes away from you to invigorate the meridians on the front of the leg. Repeat five times, bending the knee with the in-breath. Still holding the right leg, repeat the same movement, but this time stretching the heel away from you and pulling back the toes. This invigorates the meridians at the back of the leg, and particularly the important kidney and bladder points at the back of the knee (Fig. 15).

Pause before completing the movement on both sides. Rest for a few minutes, and compare the side that you have worked on to the side you have not worked on. The side you have worked on will often feel warmer and larger, a sign that there is more energy circulating. Repeat for the left leg.

Hips:

5. With the left hand under the right ankle, bring it to rest on the left thigh. If that is uncomfortable, bring the foot to the floor resting the sole of the foot on the side of the knee. Holding both the ankle and the knee and with an in-breath,

pull the knee upwards then, breathing out, push gently down towards the floor. Repeat five times with the breath. Here again it is the concentration and intention that is important not the physical movement. So even if the body cannot move very much, the energy is moving. Repeat with the left leg (Fig. 16).

6. In the same position, holding the right ankle and knee, rotate the knee five times clockwise and five times anticlockwise, allowing the right foot to move in a circle around the left knee. This sounds complicated but makes sense when you do it. The hip joints are ball-and-socket joints and need this rotation movement to keep from stiffening up. This is a difficult action, but essential in freeing the hips and groin. It works particularly on the liver and gall-bladder meridians. Repeat with the left leg (Fig. 17).

Allow the legs to stretch forward in the starting position and shake them, keeping the heels on the ground.

The groin and sexual organs:

7. Holding the feet, bring them together, soles touching, as close to the body as is comfortable. With the hands under the knees, breathe in and bring the knees together. Breathe out slowly and with the hands over the knees press gently down. Concentrate in the groin area and as you breathe out try to relax the muscles in the pelvis. This movement must be performed gently and with special awareness, as it is easy to pull the groin muscles if they are stiff. Never force and always support the knees with the hands. Repeat slowly ten times with the breath (Fig. 18).

The three yin meridians in the legs, the liver, spleen and kidneys, flow up the inside of the thigh and through the groin to join with the ren mai in the lower abdomen. Releasing tension and invigorating circulation in this area is beneficial for all three meridians, and particularly in their relation to menstruation, hernia, incontinence, etc.

If you have particular problems in this area, keep the knees apart and lie with your back and head supported by a large cushion. Allow the legs to relax completely, placing cushions under the knees if necessary. Breathe consciously and focus

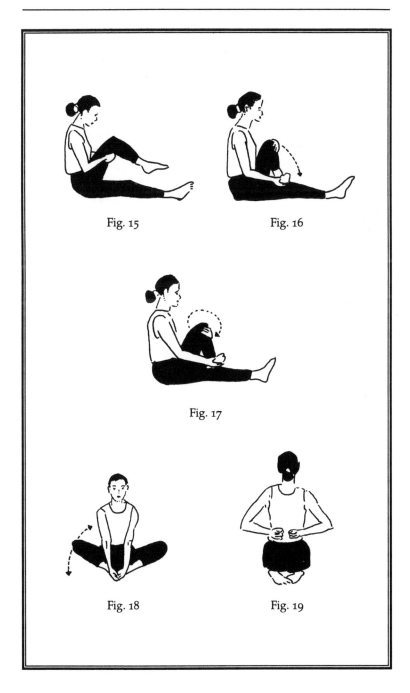

Fig. 15

Fig. 16

Fig. 17

Fig. 18

Fig. 19

your attention on relaxing and releasing tension in the pelvis. Allow your hands to rest gently over the gate of the origin (Ren 4). This position can give great relief to period pains, and in the long term help to regulate menstruation.

8. Stretch the legs forwards or sit on your heels. Rub the hands together until they feel warm. Place the hands at the back of the waist over the kidneys. Repeat three times. With a loose fist, lightly pummel the waist area either side of the spine, or if this feels too strong, rub the area with the palms of the hands. (Fig. 19).

Sit upright with the spine straight in whatever position is comfortable. Shake the hands and arms.

Hands:

9. With the arms stretched out in front of you, breathe in. Pull in the fingers making a fist with the thumb inside, held by the other fingers. As you breathe out, release the thumbs and stretch the fingers apart and away from you, imagining the qi of the meridians flowing through the fingertips (Fig. 20). Repeat ten times, co-ordinating the breath and working with the concentration. Be aware of each finger. Note any sensations.

The yin meridians in the fingers flow from the chest and along the internal aspect of the arm. They are the heart meridian which flows from the armpit through the palm of the hand to the inside of the little finger; the heart master, which flows through the palm and into the middle finger, and the lung which flows into the thumb. The yang meridians flow from the fingertips to the head and are the small intestine, which begins on the outside of the little finger, the triple heater, which begins on the ring finger, and the large intestine which flows from the index finger. They all flow along the external aspect of the arm and into the shoulders, neck and head, meeting around the eyes, nose and ears.

Wrists:

10. With the arms still stretched out in front, pull the hands alternately backwards and forwards, stretching the wrists. Try to pull back evenly, making sure that the little finger

moves as much as the thumb and index finger do. This action stimulates very important points on all six meridians in the hands, which have their source points around the wrists. Repeat ten times with the breath (Fig. 21).

11. With the elbows straight rotate the hands five times clockwise and five times anti-clockwise. You may want to rotate both hands together, but if you do each separately it is easier to concentrate and feel areas of tightness and resistance (Fig. 22).

12. Holding the left hand in the right, massage the palm with the thumb. Massage the sides of the fingers, stretching them gently. With your thumb and forefinger either side of the nail, press gently, then pull away. This again stimulates the flow of qi in the meridians (Fig. 23). Repeat for the right hand. Shake the hands and arms.

Elbows:
13. Bring the arms to shoulder level again and stretch them out in front of you. With the palms up, bring the hands to the shoulders, stretching and flexing the elbows. Repeat five times, then stretch the arms to the sides and repeat (Fig. 24).

Shoulders:
14. With the hands hanging loosely at the side, pull the shoulders up towards the ears then let them go, releasing any tension. Keep the shoulders straight, not hunching forward, or stretching back. Repeat five times. Bring the hands to the shoulders and rotate the arms, bringing the elbows together, then stretching away in as large a circle as possible. Repeat the opposite way (Fig. 25).

Shoulder massage:
15. With the right elbow loosely supported in the palm of the left hand, make a loose fist with the right hand and gently pummel the top and back of the left shoulder. Release the fist and slap the shoulders with the palm. Make sure that the elbow is well supported and the hand completely relaxed. Repeat for the opposite side (Fig. 26). Sit quietly, adjusting the position if necessary.

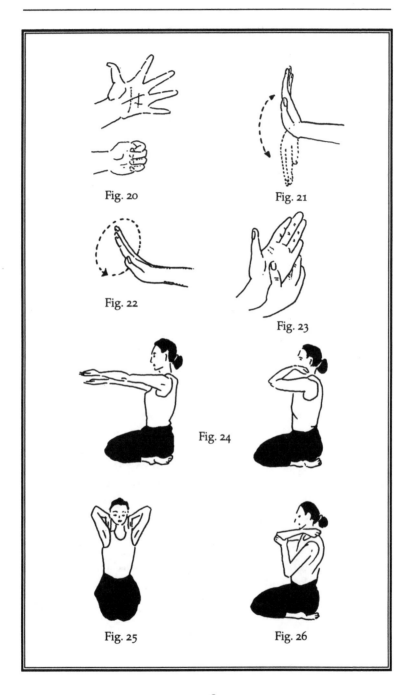

Fig. 20

Fig. 21

Fig. 22

Fig. 23

Fig. 24

Fig. 25

Fig. 26

Neck stretches:

16. With the hands relaxed in the lap, breathe quietly. Take a breath in and, exhaling, bring the chin down the chest. This should be a slow controlled movement, co-ordinated with the breath. Breathe in and return to the upright position. Breathe out as you allow the head to fall backwards. These movements should always be slow and controlled, allowing the weight of the head to stretch the muscles. Repeat for ten full breaths, five complete movements (Fig. 27).

17. Relax and take a few breaths. Breathe in and as you exhale allow the head to fall slowly to the side, bringing the ear towards the shoulder. Do not force. Breathe in as you bring the head back to the central position. Repeat on the other side. A very gentle movement is sufficient to stimulate the meridians and to relax the muscles. The neck muscles can easily be pulled if they are worked too strenuously. Repeat for ten full breaths, five complete movements (Fig. 28).

18. Relax again at the centre. Take a deep breath in. Keeping the head vertical, slowly move the head around to look over your right shoulder as you exhale. Keep the eyes wide and look around as far as you can to the back. Make sure that the top of your head remains in the centre, the neck stretches upwards as if being pulled by a rope from the top of the head, the chin is pulled slightly in. As you breathe in, slowly bring the head back to the centre. Breathe out and move slowly to the left. Repeat for ten breaths, five complete movements (Fig. 29).

Eye Massage:

19. Sitting in a relaxed position with the spine straight, rub the hands together vigorously until they are hot. Place the hands over the eyes, the centre of the palm over the centre of the eyeball. Remain still for two to three minutes with the eyes closed. Repeat three times (Fig. 30).

20. With the thumb and forefinger, pinch along the eyebrows, from the centre outwards, stimulating the points on the bladder, gall-bladder and triple-heater meridians. These points all help to revitalise the eyes and also strengthen the meridian function (Fig. 31).

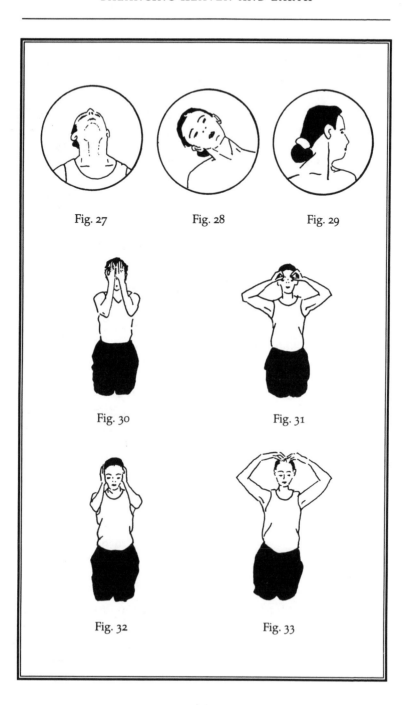

Fig. 27

Fig. 28

Fig. 29

Fig. 30

Fig. 31

Fig. 32

Fig. 33

Ear massage:
21. Rub the hands together until they are warm and place them over the ears. With the thumb and index finger pull the ear lobes, then gently squeeze around the rim of the ear.

With the hands still loosely over the ears, allow the thumbs to rest in the hollow behind the ears at the base of the skull. Keeping the shoulders relaxed, gently push the thumbs upwards. Relax and repeat, breathing out as you stretch the neck (Fig. 32).

Head massage:
22. Shake the hands with the wrist loose. Keeping the same action, lift the hands above the head, and pat the head with the fingertips, following the lines of the meridians over the head. Begin at the centre front and work slowly to the nape of the neck; gradually separate the hands and repeat, moving about an inch further from the centre line each time. If you are feeling sleepy, this will invigorate the meridians in the head and make you feel more awake (Fig. 33).

With the hands on the forehand, stroke the hair backwards, around the head, down the back of the neck, across the shoulders and down the front of the body in one long sweeping movement, as if you are brushing the body down. Repeat three times and remain sitting quietly for a few moments.

STANDING WARM-UP

For a more dynamic and energising exercise, the above sequence can be carried out in a standing position. Variations to this kind of exercise sequence are used to warm up for martial arts, tai ji and qi gong classes, and provide a simple stretch and rotation to all the joints. Thinking about the meridian flow adds another dimension and helps focus your mind on the area you are working on.

With the body relaxed, stand with the legs shoulder-width apart. Put the hands on the hips, or let them hang loosely by your side.

Feet and ankles:

1. Lift up the right foot. To the count of ten, alternately point the toes in front of you and pull them back. Although this is quite a fast movement, make sure that the toes are stretching evenly, and that the ankle is not bending to the left or right as you pull the foot back. If the foot seems to be pulling to one side, correct the movement (Fig. 34). Repeat with the left foot.

2. Turn the right foot five times clockwise, five times anti-clockwise and repeat with the left (Fig. 35).

Knees and ankles:

3. With the hands on the knees, to a count to ten, alternately bend and straighten the knees, keeping the heels on the floor. As you bend the knees, squat down as much as you can on your heels (Fig. 36); as you stretch the knees, keep the body bent forward (Fig. 37).

4. In the same position, squat down as you rotate the knees, first in a clockwise then an anti-clockwise circle (Fig. 38).

Hips:

5. Standing with the feet slightly wider than hip-width apart and the hands over the hip joints, bend the right knee while moving the weight on to the right leg. Make sure that the bent knee is centred over the toes and that the spine is straight with the tail-bone tucked under. There should be a stretch in the left hip joint (Fig. 39). Move slowly over to the left while bending the left knee (Fig. 40). Repeat the whole movement five times. This is a small movement but it produces quite a strong stretch in the hip joints, so move slowly and carefully.

6. Moving the feet slightly closer together, put the hands on the hip bones and rotate the hips around five times clockwise, five times anti-clockwise (Fig. 41).

Waist:

7. Stand straight, feet shoulder-width apart with the hands relaxed at the sides. Take a breath in and with the out-breath bend to the right side, allowing the hand to slide down the leg. Do not let the body bend forwards. With an in-breath return to the centre and with the out-breath bend to the left.

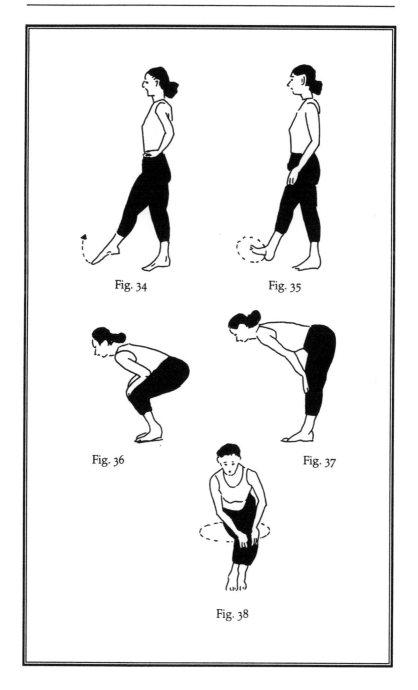

Fig. 34

Fig. 35

Fig. 36

Fig. 37

Fig. 38

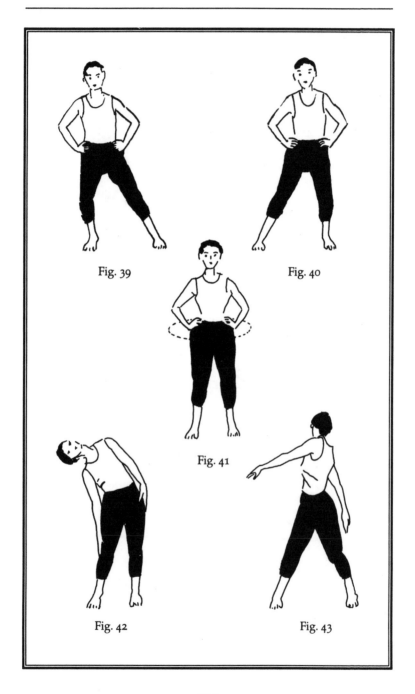

Fig. 39

Fig. 40

Fig. 41

Fig. 42

Fig. 43

Repeat for ten breaths, five times to the right, five times to the left (Fig. 42).

8. Move the feet wider apart, and with the hands by the sides, twist to the right, point with the right hand to the left foot, looking at the heel of the left foot over the shoulder. Return to the centre. Repeat to the left. Repeat the whole movement fives times (Fig. 43).

Kidneys and kidney and bladder meridians:

9. Rub the hands together until they are warm, then place them over the kidneys. Repeat three times, then rub the kidneys with the palms of the hands, or massage with a loose fist. Continue this patting movement over the centre of the buttocks and down the centre of the back of the legs, bending down and stretching the backs of the knees as you do so (Figs. 44–7).

10. Rub the hands together until they are warm; place them over the kidneys. Supporting the back waist with the hands over the kidneys, stretch back (Fig. 48).

Hands and arms:

11. With the arms stretched out in front of you, breathe in. Pull in the fingers, making a fist with the thumb inside, held by the other fingers. As you breathe out release the thumbs and stretch the fingers apart and away from you, imagining the qi of the meridians flowing through the fingertips. Repeat ten times, co-ordinating the breath and working with the concentration (Fig. 49).

12. With the hands still stretched out in front, pull the hands alternately backwards and forwards, stretching the wrists. Try to pull back evenly, making sure that the little finger moves as much as the thumb and index finger. Repeat ten times with the breath (Fig. 50).

13. With the elbows straight, rotate the hands five times clockwise and five times anti-clockwise (Fig. 51).

Elbows:

14. Bring the arms to shoulder level again and stretch them out in front of you. With the palms up, bring the hands to the

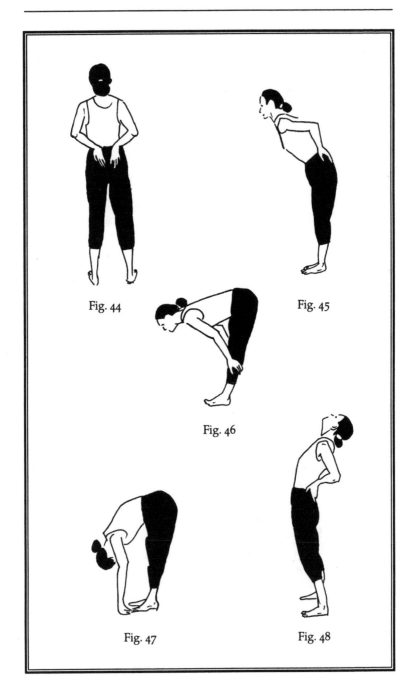

Fig. 44

Fig. 45

Fig. 46

Fig. 47

Fig. 48

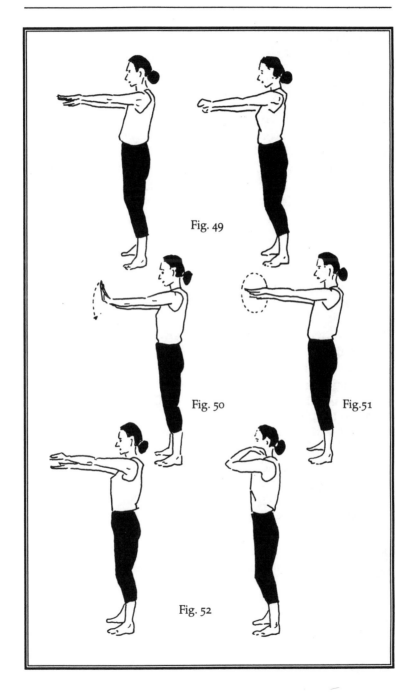

Fig. 49

Fig. 50

Fig. 51

Fig. 52

shoulders, stretching and flexing the elbows. Repeat five times, then stretch the arms to the sides and repeat (Fig. 52).

Shoulders:

15. With the hands hanging loosely at the side, pull the shoulders up towards the ears then let them go. Keep the shoulders straight, not hunching forward or stretching back. Repeat five times.

Bring the hands to the shoulders and rotate the arms, bringing the elbows together, then stretching away in as large a circle as possible. Repeat the opposite way. Ten rotations in all (Fig. 53).

Neck stretches:

16. Take a breath in and, exhaling, bring the chin down to the chest. This should be a slow, controlled movement, co-ordinated with the breath. Breathe in and return to the upright position. Breathe out as you allow the head to fall backwards. Repeat for ten full breaths, allowing the weight of the head to stretch the muscles; five complete movements (Fig. 54).

17. Relax and take a few breaths. Breathe in and as you exhale allow the head to fall slowly to the side, bringing the ear towards the shoulder. Do not force it. Breathe in as you bring the head back to the central position. Repeat on the other side. Repeat for ten full breaths, five complete movements (Fig. 55).

18. Relax again at the centre. Take a deep breath in. Keeping the head vertical, slowly move the head around to look over your right shoulder as you exhale. Keep the eyes open wide and look around as far as you can to the back. Make sure that the top of your head remains in the centre, the neck stretches upwards as if being pulled by a rope from the top of the head, the chin is pulled slightly in. As you breathe in, slowly bring the head back to the centre. Breathe out and move slowly to the left. Repeat for ten breaths, five complete movements (Fig. 56).

19. Rub the hands together and when they are warm, place them over your eyes. Repeat three times (Fig. 57).

20. Shake the hands, and when they are feeling free and loose,

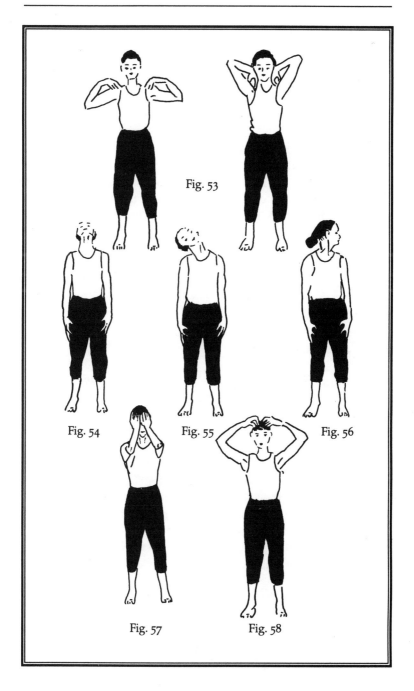

Fig. 53

Fig. 54   Fig. 55   Fig. 56

Fig. 57   Fig. 58

tap the head with the fingertips. Begin at the centre front, and work towards the back. Each time you reach the nape of the neck bring the hands back to the front and, beginning one inch from the centre line, trace three lines over the back of the head following the bladder and gall-bladder meridians (Fig. 58).

Body sweeping (Fig. 59):
Rub the hands together once more and place them over the eyes. Slowly, and with pressure, draw the hands back over the head to the nape of the neck (a), down the neck, across the shoulders and over the front of the body in one sweeping movement (b). Bring the hands round to rest on the kidneys (c), and sweep down the back of the legs (d)–(e). Repeat three times.

BALANCING LEFT AND RIGHT

SPINE STRETCHES AND TWISTS

Moving and stretching the spine is a vital part of any exercise programme. Some yoga disciplines suggest that all the various postures are aimed to correct imbalances in the spinal column and therefore to allow the correct flow of prana through the subtle channels in the spine. The importance of the centre back channel, the governor vessel, in the subtle anatomy of Chinese medicine has been discussed at length, and the bladder meridian, which flows either side of the governor vessel, contains vital points related to all the internal organs and to their nervous attachments to the spinal cord. A correctly balanced spine with all its vertebrae intact is the single most important factor in maintaining a healthy body.

For the spine to be in good shape it is not necessary to be extremely flexible. Balance and good alignment are all that are required, and much can be corrected by awareness of posture.

We all tend to stand unevenly, or have a favourite side to carry bags, shopping or children. I was so used to carrying

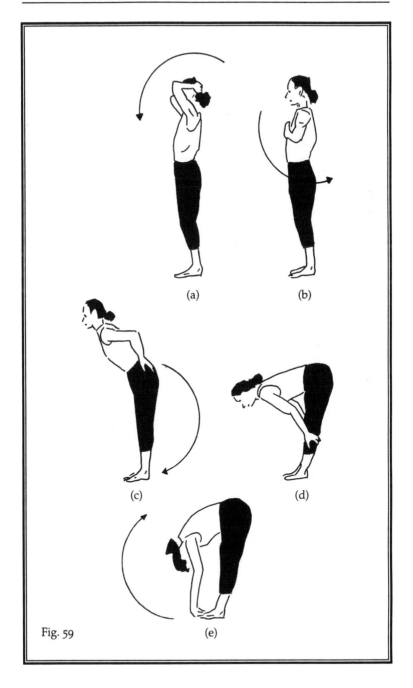

Fig. 59

(a)   (b)

(c)   (d)

(e)

my young son on my right hip that it wasn't until years later I realised that I had developed a spinal twist, very slight, but with any heavy lifting the muscles at the right of the spine began to go into spasm. This kind of thing is very common, and often can be seen on the treatment couch, with one leg appearing slightly longer than the other. In fact, one hip is raised owing to uneven muscle tension in the spine. If this situation continues it can lead to all kinds of problems – not just the obvious pain in the back but also problems in the internal organs owing to undue pressure on the nerves and subtle anatomy, and a gradual imbalance of the left and right sides of the body.

For any kind of meditation practice involving the use of the breath and concentration on the subtle energy channels and centres, exercises to correct the spine and to correct the flow of subtle energy through the spine are essential. The circulation of light breathing technique, which we will see later, helps to clear imbalances on the energetic levels, but simple spinal stretches and twists ensure that this vital area remains in good shape, allowing proper flow of blood and qi to all parts of the body.

Most of these stretches and twists are carried out on the floor. You should have something to cushion you, but this should not be too soft and spongy as you should always be aware of your body in relation to the flat surface of the floor. A thin mat or folded blanket on a wooden floor is ideal.

Preparation

Lie on your back on the floor. Allow the hands to fall away to the sides, leaving some space in the armpits. Allow the feet to fall apart. Check that the body is straight, first by looking at the position of the feet, the hips, the arms, but gradually by learning to feel. Checking your own subjective feelings against what you observe gives valuable information about your energetic imbalances and the way that your body compensates. If the spine is not balanced, we will often feel straight but in fact may be lying curved to the left or right. Lying down in a relaxed state we may also begin to feel that one side of the body is larger than the other, suggesting an imbalance of energy in the left and right sides of the body.

Take a few deep breaths, allowing the body to relax. Feel the weight of the pelvis on the floor and check that the hips feel level, and that the weight is evenly distributed between the left and the right. Relax the lower back. The natural curve of the spine means that the lower back does not usually touch the floor but, with relaxation of the muscles in this area, the spine gradually relaxes and releases. If you feel any pain or discomfort in the lower back, bring the feet towards the buttocks and lie with the knees up. This should release tension in the lower spine.

Bring your attention to the upper back and shoulder blades. Allow the back to sink into the floor. Allow the shoulder blades to move downwards and inwards, opening the chest and keeping the shoulders down. This is a subtle movement which can be performed in the imagination if the body is not sure what to do. Check that the head is straight.

For more extended periods of relaxation or for breathing exercises, the head should be supported on a book or folded blanket. If using a blanket, bring it right down to your shoulders so that the neck can be completely supported. Allow the arms to roll outwards, opening the armpits and turning the palms upwards.

In this position the yin meridians are all exposed, the yang is made quiet. By turning the arms out in this way, the heart and lung meridians flowing from the chest through the armpits and into the palms of the hands are opened out, bringing calm and tranquillity and allowing maximum effi-ciency of the chest and lungs. But this is a position of vulnerability, and care must be taken that you do not get cold. If intending to remain in the position for some time cover yourself with a light blanket.

This is the basic prone position, and as with the basic standing and sitting positions, we will come back to it again and again. Much can be done lying down, and if you are forced to be in bed, or are too lacking in energy to move around, you do not have to be totally inactive; there is much to be done with the breath, with the concentration and with subtle body movements.

Spine stretches:
1. Take a couple of deep breaths to come out of your relaxed state. Bring the feet together. With the arms stretched out on the floor behind you, take a breath in and, as you breathe out, stretch the body, concentrating on the hands and feet and feeling the fingers and toes stretching evenly in opposite directions. Relax as you breathe in. Repeat a few times (Fig. 60).

Repeat a further three times stretching the heels and pulling up the toes. This gives more stimulation to the kidney, bladder and gall-bladder meridians.

Feel as you stretch that the energy is moving through the meridians and coursing out through the end points at the tips of the fingers and toes. As you breathe in, imagine drawing energy back to the centre.

2. Roll over on to the abdomen, with the arms stretched out in front of you. Breathe in and stretch the hands forwards and upwards, bringing the head away from the floor, and looking up with the eyes. Breathe in and relax. Take a few breaths. Repeat three times (Fig. 61).

3. Inhale deeply, and with the exhalation stretch the feet and legs away from the body, bringing them as far as possible off the floor. This may only be an inch or so, but it creates the correct action in the spine. Do not force it and do not hold for longer than the out-breath. Make sure that the breath is stable before you repeat. Repeat three times (Fig. 62).

4. Breathe in, and on an exhalation stretch the right arm and the right leg, keeping the head on the floor; repeat three times. Then repeat with the left side (Fig. 63).

Rest with the head turned to the side; take a few deep breaths. Inhale and with an exhalation stretch the right arm and the left leg, while the left arm and right leg remain completely relaxed. Repeat three times. Then repeat by stretching the left arm and right leg.

5. Inhale deeply, and with the exhalation stretch the hands

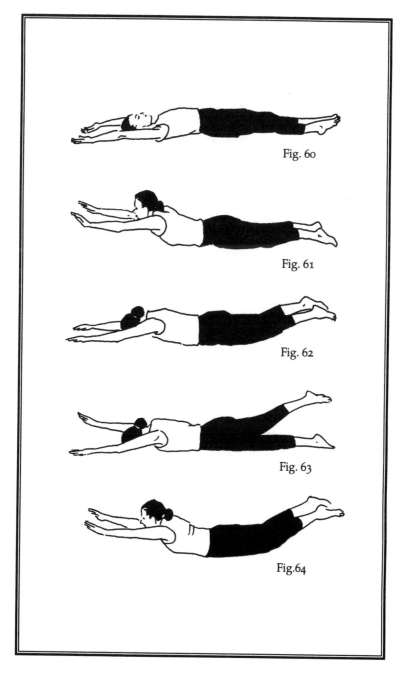

Fig. 60

Fig. 61

Fig. 62

Fig. 63

Fig.64

and feet away from the body, bringing them as far away from the floor as possible. Do not hold for longer than the exhalation. Take a few even breaths and completely relax before the next stretch. Repeat three times (Fig. 64).

These simple stretches help to adjust the meridian flow in the upper and lower and left and right sides of the body. If there is any pain or discomfort in the lower back, roll over on to your back and bring your knees to your chest.

6. Remaining in the same position, bring the hands to the sides of the shoulders, palms and forehead on the floor. Take a breath in. As you breathe out, slowly move the head upwards, allowing the nose and then the chin to come in contact with the floor; continue the backward movement of the head, allowing the eyes to lead. Stretching the front of the neck, bring the shoulders and chest off the floor; the weight is taken by the hands and the lower abdomen, which remains in contact with the floor. Look up to the ceiling and imagine that you can see down the wall behind you to the floor. The movement should take the time of the exhalation, but can be broken just before the shoulders come off the floor with another in-breath if necessary. Breaking the movement allows you to slow down and give more time to experience the full sensation of the stretch. Repeat three times (Fig. 65).

7. Lying on the back with the arms stretched along the floor behind the head, take a few deep breaths (Fig. 66). After the third exhalation, inhale as you bring the arms over the head. As the hands move forward over the head allow them to pull the body erect until you are sitting up with the arms stretching forwards. Exhale, moving the body forwards over the legs, reaching with the hands for the feet and ankles. Relax in this forward bend as you fully exhale (Fig. 67). This should become one smooth fluid movement.

Inhaling, gradually sit up and, exhaling, lie back and extend the arms back over the head. Move slowly and carefully, imagining each vertebra as it comes in contact with the floor (Fig. 68).

Repeat as often as is comfortable. Create your own rhythm

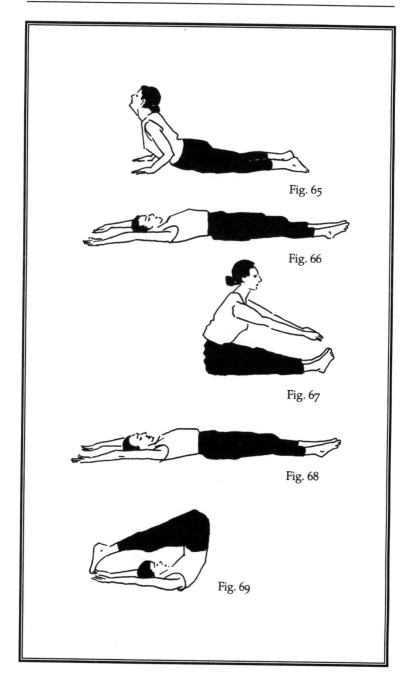

Fig. 65

Fig. 66

Fig. 67

Fig. 68

Fig. 69

of breathing and moving, not overstretching or straining, but allowing your weight gradually to move the body further forward.

8. If this movement is easy for you, carry it further. As your body reaches its resting position on the floor, lift the legs over the head and down towards the fingertips on the floor behind the head (Fig. 69). Put the two movements together and create a rhythmic wavelike pattern. Speeded up, this movement is actually much easier as your momentum draws you into the next position. It's good to try different speeds and see how they feel. Very slowly, you can pay attention to each vertebra as the spine curls and uncurls on the floor.

Spinal twists:
1. Lying on your back with the hands on the abdomen, bring the knees up until the feet are as close as possible to the buttocks. Breathe evenly and allow the muscles in the back to relax (Fig. 70). Stretch the arms horizontally to the sides.

Inhale and, with an exhalation, let the knees drop to the right, keeping both shoulders firmly on the floor. Look to the left. Inhale and return the knees to the centre. Repeat to the left, looking to the right (Fig. 71). Repeat three times.

2. Move the feet off the ground until the thighs are vertical, and repeat the above movements. This works on the area around the waist and stimulates the kidneys (Fig. 72).

3. Move the knees further forward, to an angle of about 60°, and repeat the exercise. This works on the middle thoracic spine and the diaphragm, and stimulates the digestive organs.

4. For a stronger stretch, lie with the legs stretched out in front and the arms in their horizontal position. Bring the left foot to the right knee, and the right hand to the left knee. Inhale, and exhale as you look to the left and use the right hand to bring the left knee towards the floor. Do not force but allow the weight of the leg gradually to bring the knee closer to the floor, keeping the shoulders in contact with the floor at all times. This is a wonderful stretch, especially when performed with a long, slow exhalation. When you have reached the extent of your stretch, breathe quietly, trying to relax and

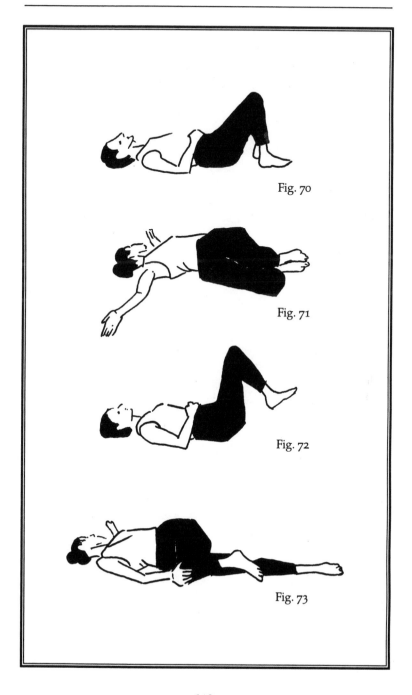

Fig. 70

Fig. 71

Fig. 72

Fig. 73

release further with each exhalation. Take your time. Repeat on the opposite side (Fig. 73).

These simple spinal stretches and twists do wonders for the whole body and vitality. Once the energy is flowing well in the spine, so much internal imbalance can begin to correct itself. The twists, if carried out frequently, can help to remedy displaced vertebrae and spinal misalignments. A healthy, supple spine is the foundation of good health, physically, mentally and emotionally. The yang energy of the governor vessel (du mai) is able to warm, invigorate and penetrate all the vital centres along the spine, bringing warmth and vitality to the sexual organs and the digestive organs, rhythmic movement and clarity to the lungs and the heart, and the light of the spirits to the brain and sensory organs.

QI GONG FOR BALANCING THE RIGHT AND LEFT SIDES OF THE BODY

Standing in the basic qi gong position, feet parallel and hip-width apart, knees relaxed, feel the feet in contact with the floor, with even weight on the right and left foot, on the heels and the balls of the feet, and on the inside and outside of the soles of the feet. Spend a few minutes feeling this contact. Imagine the feet are your roots, keeping you stable and balanced, and bringing cooling, moistening yin energy from the earth.

Let the upper body relax, with the arms hanging loosely at the sides. Bring the attention to the point at the top of the head, and from this point feel as if you are being pulled upwards, the neck and spine gently elongating.

If you find this difficult to imagine, put the palms of the hands over the tops of the ears, so that the middle fingers meet at the centre of the top of the head. From this point, take a large, even strand of hair and pull gently upwards. Imagine that you are suspended from this point; the chin naturally moves inward, the neck stretches, and the whole of the spine is able to align itself to the centre.

From this point imagine a section being drawn through the centre of the body, following the line of the spine and the centre front (the pathways of the governor vessel and the conception vessel), so that the body is cut in half. Make the line completely straight, as if a sheet of glass has been placed between the left and right sides of the body.

Be aware of any differences you are feeling in the left and right, and make small adjustments in your position to correct these differences as much as possible. As you feel the two sides of the body becoming more even, imagine the space between the left and right widening, as if this central space is filled with nothing but pure energy. Breathe naturally, allowing the breath to merge with the empty space through your centre.

BREATHING EXERCISES

THE DAOIST CIRCULATION OF LIGHT

This exercise fulfils the function of clearing and balancing all the energy centres in a similar way to the basic qi gong exercise, but it uses only the breath and the concentration. The more physical the exercise, the more obviously physical the effect. By using the breath and by concentrating the mind we are not affecting the muscles in the same way as with physical movement, but we are stimulating the subtle energy flow, and therefore balancing the flow of energy in the meridians and affecting the function of the internal organs. All the internal organs have direct connections via the nervous system to the spine; and either side of the spine all the internal organs have their main acupuncture points. Working with the central spine channel is therefore the most effective way to balance the body's subtle energy system.

The circulation of the light exercise uses the extraordinary meridians, the governor vessel (du mai) in the spine, and the conception vessel (ren mai) on the centre front to create balance in all the internal organs and the three burning spaces.

Method:
Sit comfortably, on a chair, on the floor with the legs crossed (Fig. 74) or on a pad with the legs folded backwards (Fig. 75).

It is important that the spine is straight and it should not be supported. If it is difficult to sit with crossed legs with the knees on the floor, it is better to assume one of the other positions, as it is important in all sitting meditation that the posture is stable and the spine is straight. If you are sitting on a chair, place the feet evenly on the ground and be aware of the contact between the feet and the floor (Fig. 76). Feel that the body weight is even on the buttocks. Fold your hands together in your lap, or place them on your knees. For this exercise your palms should be facing in towards the body rather than upwards. Various hand movements and mudras create different energetic impulses, and for this exercise all needs to be turned within.

Close your eyes and turn the attention to the breath. Breath naturally and slowly.

1. Bring the awareness to the lower tip of the spine and imagine a light shining there. Breathe in and out a few times, slightly contracting the pelvic floor muscles as you breathe in, letting them go as you breathe out.

2. When you are able to visualise or imagine a light, breathe in deeply, imagining the light travelling up the spine, through the gate of life (du mai 4, Plate 4) at the level of the waist, past the way of the spirits (du mai 11) at the level of the heart, through the back of the neck and over the top of the head to rest between the eyebrows.

3. Pause for a few seconds with the breath held, then breathe out, slowly bringing the light through the centre front line of the ren mai (Plate 5), through the centre of the chest (ren mai 17), the centre of the upper abdomen (ren mai 12) and then down through the navel to the sea of qi (ren mai 6) and the gate of origin (ren mai 4).

This is one circulation (Fig. 77).

Variations:

If it is difficult to attain one circulation with one breath, stop at certain points on the way. In time you will feel areas that may benefit from further attention, but at first try pausing at the centre of the back, at the level of the heart and the acupuncture point the way of the spirits. Breathe out, releas-

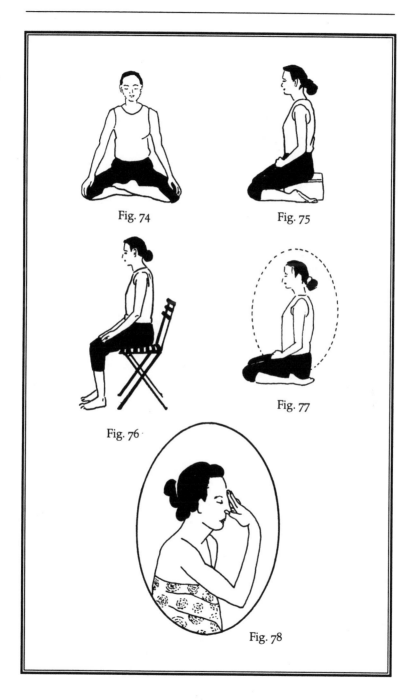

Fig. 74

Fig. 75

Fig. 76

Fig. 77

Fig. 78

ing any tension in the area and, as you breathe in, resume your inner journey upwards towards the brow centre. Here, pause again, breathe out and in again a few times, concentrating the breath between the eyebrows. Feel that you are breathing in and out through this centre. Take a breath in, and breathing out bring the light through the centre front line, stopping again to take a few breaths at the heart centre if it feels more comfortable. When the breath is fully exhaled, concentrate for a few seconds on the lower abdomen before beginning a new cycle.

Try ten slower circulations, followed by ten faster circulations, keeping in mind the function of the ren mai and du mai as the primary yin yang channels (see p. 69). As your breath becomes stronger and longer, the circulation will become slower and easier.

Benefits:
This exercise is often used as a preliminary balancing technique before any deeper concentration or meditation is attempted. By concentrating on this primary yin/yang circulation, we are working on our imbalances and instabilities, harmonising the qi, and aiding the meridian flow and organ function. We all tend to over-use one centre, or have specific weaknesses in a particular internal organ. The circulation of light exercise is a very safe way to address these fundamental imbalances, and a particularly safe way to enter the world of meditation if you are practising alone. My Japanese meditation teacher always advised a ten-minute practice of the circulation of light as a preparation for any more advanced concentration techniques. And during times of physical or emotional stress this would often be the only practice performed.

Concentration exclusively to one centre, whether it be the hara, the heart or the brow centre, may cause problems if not done with awareness. As we become more aware of the needs of our body we are more able to decide which practice is most suitable. But if we are in any doubt, the circulation of light is always safe and very effective.

Both the Indian yoga and the Daoist traditions mention an

alternative method of imagining that the breath is being taken in through the heels. This also suggests a connection with the yin and yang qiao mai, which have their joint beginnings in the heels.

ALTERNATE NOSTRIL BREATHING

Although not strictly part of the Chinese tradition, instructions for alternate nostril breathing are given here as it is a very useful and effective way of balancing the energy in the left and right sides of the body, and also to clear the nose and the airways. If one nostril is permanently blocked, this is bound to affect the rest of the energtic system.

Method:
Sitting in a comfortable position with the spine straight (see suggested positions for the circulation of light, Figs 74–6). With the hands resting on the knees, relax the body, concentrating only on the body and the breath.

Bring the right hand to the face, placing the thumb over the right nostril, the ring finger over the left nostril. The second and third fingers rest giving slight pressure to the eyebrow centre. Alternatively, each finger rests in the depression at the internal end of the eyebrows (acupuncture point Bladder 2), stimulating the bladder meridian and the yin and yang qiao mai. The second and third fingers do not move throughout the practice (Fig. 78).

Close the right nostril with the thumb. Breathe in through the left nostril to a slow count of five. Close the left nostril with the fourth finger. Release the right nostril and breathe out through the right nostril to a slow count of five. Breathe in through the right nostril, then place the thumb on the right nostril, release the left nostril and breathe out through the left. This is one cycle.

It is important that the in- and out-breath are regular, without noise and with an even count. Be aware of the feeling of the breath on the nostrils. The number of the counting can vary according to what feels comfortable, increasing the number of the count as you become more practised. If there is any feeling of discomfort, shorten the length of the breath, never force or hold the breath.

Advanced method:
After breathing in and with both nostrils closed, count slowly to five before breathing out. The count is now: breathe in for five, retain breath for five, breathe out for five. This variation should only be performed once the first stage has been practised regularly. Although these methods are simple, they are very effective and care should always be taken to do only that which is natural and comfortable. As always, learn to look within and listen to the body. The body should become calm, the mind passive. If there is any agitation, palpitations or feelings of anxiety, the practice should be discontinued. Take a few steady, natural breaths, and try the practice again without holding the breath. The process of balancing the subtle body energies is a delicate one and can never be achieved by force.

PART 4

WORKING WITH
THE FIVE ELEMENTS

Practical Ways to Strengthen
Your Particular Weakness

THE FIRE ELEMENT AND THE HEART

Fire is associated with mid-summer; it is yang in nature and relates to heat. Its natural movement is the upward movement of fire. It therefore needs to remain cool and grounded. It is the role of the heart in the body to rule the other organs; the beat of the heart gives rhythm to all the subtle autonomic functions and the circulation of the blood brings nutrition and oxygen to every cell. Being yang in nature, the fire element does not like too much heat or movement, and will react by becoming too yang – too excitable, too hot, too fast. An imbalance of fire in the body will manifest in these same ways, creating such symptoms as heat, agitation, insomnia, palpitations, mental confusion, speediness. The face may easily become red and flushed.

Each organ reacts to an extreme of its own climate and the heart may be damaged by an excess of heat, but the organs also can be damaged by an excess of their associated emotion, and with the heart the emotion is joy. It is difficult to imagine being harmed by joy, but here there is the suggestion of over-excitement, over-stimulation which puts too much pressure on the heart. We saw in Part 1 that there are two types of joy associated with the heart, one which is often translated as excitement, the other as a calm, peaceful joy. Joy is literally the feeling of our hearts being lifted, a kind of *joie de vivre*, or the joy of being alive. The spirit that resides in the heart needs to be in contact with heaven, and it is this contact that creates joy in our lives. In meditation we hope to make this connection with heaven, or the connection with our higher selves and achieve a feeling of light-heartedness and peace.

As each organ suffers from an excess of its natural movements, so it can also suffer from a repression of that natural movement. And the heart can be damaged by a lack of joy, particularly if this is a long-term depression.

We all know that even if we have times of experiencing deep joy, it can be easily lost. In times of depression our relationship to heaven is obscured, as clouds obscure the sun. And it can be helpful to think of this darkness as caused by clouds. They come and go. Observe them and try to find out what makes them, always aiming to remember that even when the sky is grey, the sun is still there, and most important that the clouds are of our own making.

The ancient Chinese classics, both Daoist and Confucian, describe these clouds as being made from our attachments and desires. It is only human to experience emotions and desires, but the clouds begin to form when the mind becomes preoccupied by a particular emotion, or possessed by a desire that is not in alignment with our own true destiny or our own true nature. Meditation can give us a chance to break through those clouds – if only momentarily – and to see things as they really are. Over-emphasis on any one emotion tends to be the result of not accepting the reality of our present situation, either wanting things to be as they were or wishing for things to be other than they are. But it is only through an acceptance of our present situation that we are able to move forward.

Even in the most dire situations of life we must remember that we are in control, that we have made our lives and that we have the power to make them different. And if we cannot change the external circumstances, then we can change our attitude to them.

Our experience tells us that the amount of joy in our lives has very little to do with external circumstances, yet we all tend to think that everything will be all right if ..., things will be much better when ..., whereas joy is the acceptance of life as it is, not with a passive resignation to fate, but an ability to be here, now – based in the reality of the present but with a willingness to change and grow according to the circumstances of our lives and in accordance with our own true nature.

RITUAL

Joy is the natural emotion of the heart, and ritual is the associated 'virtue'. In traditional societies, ritual plays a central role in daily and yearly life, giving the individual a sense of being part of a greater order. When I lived in Japan I embraced the rituals of the culture and the rituals of the various Shinto and Buddhist temples where I trained. At the martial arts dojo we bowed to the pictures of the founders, greeted each other and our teachers with formal gestures. In the temples we washed our hands at a particular water fountain, in a particular way, sat facing a certain direction and never allowed our feet to point towards the altar.

When walking in the countryside we would pass small wayside shrines, and place a flower or a small stone, giving a prayer of thanks for the protection of the various nature spirits and deities. And even in the centre of the cities, at every corner there would be a reminder of the presence of the gods, and the chance to take a few minutes' break from the chaos of the city to light some incense or pull the huge rope in front of the Shinto shrine, to ring the bell and alert any local spirits of your presence. To me this was like becoming a child again, allowing myself to play, to talk to the invisible. It was fun. But it came about from a deep respect for nature and for the unknown. And it was an effective way to keep in touch with the wonder and joy of life.

Returning to the West I attempted to import some of the Eastern rituals, but that didn't feel right. Each place demands its own rituals, and we in the West have successfully removed most of ours. It has taken me a long time to accept the fact that I can invent my own.

RITUAL FOR THE FOUR SEASONS

The most fundamental rituals in any society are those marking the seasonal progression of the year. And this is the simplest and most effective way to begin if we wish to reintroduce ritual into our lives. Each tradition celebrates the solstices to mark the longest and shortest days and the equinoxes to mark the times of equilibrium. March 21st marks the manifestation of spring, when life can be observed breaking through from the cold of winter and when the return of life and growth is celebrated. Spring-cleaning is an appropriate ritual at this time of year, throwing open windows and doors that have remained closed in the winter, opening up, airing out; and as with our homes, so with the rest of our lives. Spring is a time to stretch ourselves, take on new projects, do more exercise; it is an outward-looking, expansive time.

We can mark the spring equinox by filling our rooms with spring flowers, moving furniture, creating change. Traditionally in Japan, different types of flower would be used in arrangements at different times of the year, obviously dictated by availability; but not only the flowers would change, the calligraphy and paintings would also be changed with each season to mark the progression of the year, and in a more subtle way to reflect the different energy of each season.

In Heian times, possibly the height of ritual society in Japan, courtiers would dress in different colours to reflect the different seasonal energies, wearing blues and greens in the spring, reds and yellows in the summer, purples and white in the autumn, and dark blue and black in the winter. This might be in the form of an undergarment only – but according to the Chinese tradition, each of these colours resonates with the energies of the season and with the associated organ. Using those colours in ritual is another way to tune in with the natural cycles of the year, and an aid to healing.

As spring is the time for expansion and movement, new projects and ideas, so summer is the time for fruition and creativity. The summer solstice is the time when we are in contact with heaven, closest to the sun. Midsummer rituals

162

are sun rituals, creativity rituals. We can watch nature ripen and flower and begin to form fruit. The summer solstice is the time when we are most open, most able to be in contact with heaven and the spirits, most able to be our true creative, expressive selves. But the Chinese medical classics always warn against going too far, advising us to take care not to over-extend, not to float away.

Summer is the time of the splendour of the flower, but autumn is the time of the fruit. The autumn equinox, the time of the harvest festival and the celebration of the fruits of the earth, is always tinged with the sadness of the end of summer. But the celebration of the harvest serves to remind us that for the fruit to mature and ripen the flower has to die. And to remain constantly open to heaven is not to bear fruit in the world. Autumn is a time of restriction, of cutting back, of getting rid of what is unnecessary in order to survive the winter. It is a time of letting go of what is no longer useful, letting go of things, ideas, projects, anything that is taking up too much of our time and energy and not bearing fruit. As much as spring is a time to be open and embrace the world, so autumn is a time of closing down, weighing things up, being selective; just as the wheat is separated from the chaff after the harvest we need to keep what is of value and discard what is not.

This is a time of preparation for winter, when energies are focused inward. In winter we eat warm food; the energy must be conserved, guarding against cold. The winter solstice marks the time of the least sun, the least contact with heaven. Many of the ancient ritual sites for the winter solstice were in caves, marking the descent into the earth and the ritual descent into the underworld. The winter solstice is a time of ritual death, the death of the old to make way for the new. Unless the seed is frozen deep within the earth in winter it may not make a good, strong plant in the spring. The time of mid-winter, of cold, dark and withdrawal of the sun, should be marked by a similar ritual. It is a time of deep inner contemplation, meditation and stillness; the time when we can become most easily silent and stable. At the summer solstice we could have easy access to heaven, but winter is a time when many people feel cut off, low in energy and in spirit. This time can be used for stillness, for a sense of oneness with the earth and the qualities of yin. This is a time when we need to light candles, burn incense, keep the fire alive in the depths of winter, as the fire of the gate of life enlivens the yin of the kidneys, bringing the spark of new life.

At its best, ritual can bring us in touch with the spirtual aspect of our being, helping us to maintain a balance between heaven and earth and to acknowledge the cycles of nature. At its worst, ritual can become restrictive – a strait-jacket in which there is no room for personal expression and the actions no longer have power. Rather than adopt rituals that have outgrown their usefulness or lost their meaning through the centuries, try creating your own rituals that speak to the soul. Begin by lighting a candle and burning natural oils when you take a bath to ensure that it is a time of pleasure and relaxation, a time to tune in to your body and to visualise your healing. Progress to making your own shrine from things that you love – things that remind you of beauty and keep you in touch with your aspirations. Change your shrine regularly, possibly with the change of seasons, to remind yourself that you are in the process of change and growth and have different needs at different times. Marking the yearly festivals can help us to remain in contact with nature and the constant cycles of change and transformation. To the ancient Chinese, adhering to the cycles of nature was called 'following the way to heaven'.

EXERCISES FOR THE HEART

The heart requires calming and cooling, quiet and regularity, joy and contact with heaven. Insomnia, palpitations, hypertension, and even mania will all respond to breathing exercises and meditation, and this is the best way to remain in touch with heaven, to regulate the mind and the emotions and to keep in touch with the natural joy of life. Meditation is the safest and most traditional way to approach all heart imbalances. If the heart is calm, relaxed and joyful, the rest of the body will respond, just as in ancient times when the emperor was strong and calm, the empire was peaceful.

It is often the stillness of the body that draws attention to the activity of the mind. But in stilling the body we can also begin to still the mind, by observing but not engaging. And we can work on this while walking down the street, waiting for the bus, and in any other activity, by consciously bringing the mind back to the present, back to the task at hand; to be aware of the breath and centred in the body.

Standing qi gong

Stand in the basic qi gong position with the hands on the lower abdomen (Fig. 79). Take a few deep breaths and concentrate the mind. As you inhale, bring the hands to the centre of the chest, the fingers facing the midline (Fig. 80). Breathe out, stretching the arms out at shoulder height, visualising the pathway of the heart meridian, flowing from deep within the chest and emerging in the armpit, along the lower, inside face of the arm, into the palm and little finger. Imagine breath flowing out through the little finger (Fig. 81).

Remain in this position breathing naturally for a few moments then bring the hands back to the lower abdomen and repeat the movement. Allow your body to find its own rhythm, experimenting with the breath and with the visualisation until you have achieved a movement that feels natural.

The meridians of the heart and heart master (pericardium) both flow into the palm of the hand (Ht8 and HM8), and it is this movement of energy from the chest to the palm that provides the energetic impulse for hand healing to be performed. The other two meridians connected with the fire element, the triple burner and the small intestine, also flow in the arms and the hands, the little finger containing both the 'emperor' fire meridians, the heart and the small intestine. Tony Agpaoa, one of the psychic surgeons of the Philippines, demonstrated many times in public that he could cut through several layers of tape with the energy emitted from his little finger. When I watched the early Philippine healers at work,

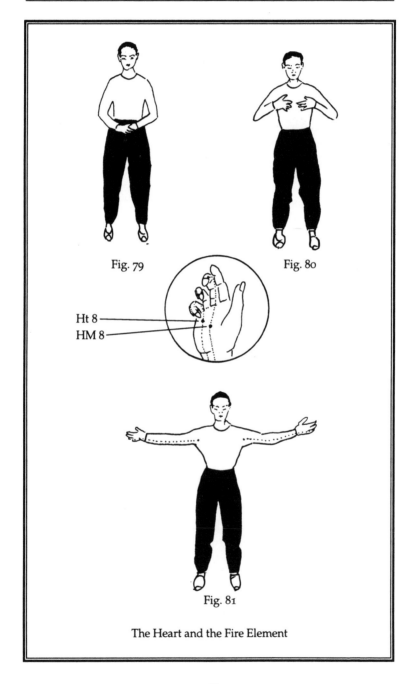

Fig. 79

Fig. 80

Ht 8
HM 8

Fig. 81

The Heart and the Fire Element

many of them used their little fingers to penetrate into the tissues of the body. This kind of control over subtle energy is obviously very rare, but all healers have this same ability in varying degrees, and we can all learn to access it to heal ourselves. In performing this simple exercise and visualisation we stimulate the healing energy by activating the heart meridian and also encourage a healthy flow of energy to the chest and heart.

Conclude the exercise by gathering energy back to the chest and placing the hands over the heart – a gesture or mudra that symbolises humility and protects the heart centre. Humility is a necessary quality for all healers; it prevents us from doing too much and assuming we can be all things to all people. It reminds us that we are only human and that when we are working with others, we must also remember to take care of ourselves. This mudra can help the healer restore her own energy.

Meditation

All meditation is beneficial for the heart, but particularly regulation of the breathing and simple counting techniques which train the mind to empty itself of unwanted thoughts and distractions. Far Eastern traditions stress that the heart must be empty and calm for the spirit to manifest, and images such as the still, calm pool are often used in visualisation. Visualisations for the heart chakra in Indian yoga will often use the image of a lotus flower floating in a vast lake. In each case the essence is of a calm expanse, in which each thought may cause a ripple, but if left alone the pool will become calm again.

Regulating the breath and the rhythm of the heart

Sitting comfortably with the back straight (or lying down if necessary) focus the mind on the breath. Make sure that the armpits are slightly open and that the arms are not too close to the sides of the body; feel that the chest has plenty of space to expand sideways, and that air can circulate freely. Placing the hands with the palms upwards on the knees or in the lap naturally brings the arms into the correct position. Relax the shoulders. Feel the air as it moves gently through the nostrils, the gentle expansion and contraction of the ribcage. Concentrating the mind completely on the breath, begin counting slowly to four with each inhalation, and to four with each exhalation. Repeat for five minutes.

If you feel breathless at any time, stop, take a few deep breaths and when the breath is totally calm, continue. When discussing breathing exercises for the lungs we will go further with this exercise, increasing the count and changing the ratio of counts between inhalation and exhalation, but to help the heart and to bring rhythm and regularity to the heart centre this simple exercise is all that is required. Any straining or holding the breath will not help calm the heart but give added strain, and that is not the aim here. Think of each breath as a wave in a calm sea as it washes over the beach, each new wave adding to the endless rhythm of the ebb and flow of the tide. These are the rhythms of nature and our bodies need to be in touch with those rhythms; the heart centre and the upper heater give rhythm to all the deep functions of the body, from the movement of food through the passages of the alimentary canal to the opening and closing of the pores. The heart in its position as emperor of the body co-ordinates all this, and it can do so with rhythm and ease or with stress and irregularity.

One of the main obstacles to achieving this kind of peaceful rhythm in the heart is boredom. Our bodies love rhythms, our minds enjoy change and excitement. Calming the mind will help to give you the patience to stay with it – to keep at it even if you feel you are doing nothing. As with so much subtle exercise, it is not the sudden dramatic changes that are important but the slow, quiet rhythmic movements that create permanent change, as the sea eventually erodes the land, the drip of water makes a hole through the stone.

Calming the mind by counting the breath

Sitting in a comfortable position with the back straight, focus the attention on the breath. Be aware of your in-breath and out-breath without trying to change it; as you relax, it will naturally become slightly slower and deeper.

Begin counting your breaths, one cycle of inhalation and exhalation to each count, from one to ten. Then begin again. Repeat for five minutes, which, depending on the length of your breath, may be two or three cycles. Allow thoughts to come and go, observe them but do not engage in conversation with them, and always try to keep to the count, keep to the breath. If you find that you have followed a thought and lost the count just begin again. It is the trying, rather than the perfection that brings results. Don't get angry with yourself if your mind wanders – some days will be good, some will be bad; try not to engage the emotions in judging yourself a success or failure. Just do the practice.

When working with the heart centre we must try to develop a mixture of humility and self-love: being nice to ourselves, owning and accepting our weakesses, not expecting perfection. Coming out of a meditation exercise thinking how useless we are because we didn't manage to get to ten once in ten minutes is not going to do much good. Learn to laugh about it, but carry on. Tomorrow will be different, and if it isn't, then maybe the next, or the next. The important thing is to keep on through the good days and the bad days without judgement. Just sit. Just breathe. And just count.

Gradually increase the time to ten minutes, and if you want to engage in a more serious practice finally to twenty. Twenty minutes is often the minimum recommended time for a meditation to have deep changing results, though any period of concentrated breathing will have beneficial effects on the body.

A regular daily practice of sitting and breathing for twenty minutes can bring about remarkable changes in our state of mind and our ability to deal with stress. Once you have tried the various exercises suggested, you can make your own practice, possibly with ten minutes of circulation of light, to balance yin and yang and clear the subtle energy channels, and ten minutes of counting the breath; or ten minutes of counting the in- and out-breaths followed by ten minutes of quiet concentration on the hara or heart centre. It is important to try out what feels right, as different techniques are more suitable for different people, and different techniques more suitable for each of us at different times.

If you are speedy and are finding it difficult to sleep, concentrate on the lower abdomen. If you need mental invigoration, concentrate on the centre between the eyebrows. If you need to balance the two, concentrate on the heart centre, visualising a deep pool of clear blue-green water, each thought just a ripple on the pool. Watch the ripples spreading out and fading away.

THE WATER ELEMENT AND THE KIDNEYS

The water element is associated with mid-winter, with darkness, with the interior and with cold. Its energy is yin and descends. The kidneys govern the water in the body, the lower abdomen, fertility and life cycles. They are responsible for the deepest of the bodily energies and reserves and are particularly harmed by overwork. Any long-term depletion from overwork or illness will ultimately affect the kidneys. The kidneys are also said to store the inherited, constitutional energies, so many deep-seated problems may surface with kidney-type symptoms. If the kidneys are weak, the body tends to feel cold, especially in the lower back and along the spine, and in the lower abdominal area. There can be general tiredness, and stiffness in the lower back. The teeth and hair may be weak.

One of the simplest and yet most important things to do to help the kidneys is to keep them warm. In Japan many people can still be seen in winter wearing the traditional 'haramaki' – a band of soft, light wool worn over the kidneys and protecting the vital points on the spine and at the centre of the lower abdomen. This ensures that these vital energy points are protected from cold, and if this area of our central furnace – the basis of our metabolism and energy production – is kept warm, the whole body is able to feel warm. We have seen that the kidney meridian flows through the sole of the foot and is the only meridian to have direct contact with the earth. Cold can enter the kidney meridian through the feet, and it is therefore important to keep the feet warm. Coldness contracts, which then causes the whole system of communication to contract – the blood is not getting through, and neither is the qi.

A patient with long-term Chronic Fatigue Syndrome experienced her greatest step towards recovery when she began actively to keep herself warm. She was so cut off from her body-knowing by years of repression and more recently by the weight she had gained below her waist, that she was unable to recognise that she was cold. As she began to wear more clothes, and in fact knit herself a 'haramaki', she realised that since her early childhood, spent in an inhospitable girls' boarding school, she had repressed her feelings of cold. She was in fact frozen. She had no doubt gained the weight as an attempt by her body to protect this vital centre, but the fire of alchemical transmutation in the lower abdomen had all but gone out, and her energy production was almost at a standstill. On each of her visits to the clinic I had used warming treatments with moxa on her lower back, but it was not until she was able to tune into her own resources and begin to nurture herself that she began to make real progress.

The kidneys are obviously more at danger in the winter months, and particular care should be taken to keep the body warm at this time. The older we are, the more we need to pay attention to the lower abdominal area, protecting it from cold, stimulating it with massage and keeping the lower spine flexible with exercises. In winter we should eat warming foods: roots and pulses, soups and stews, leaving salads and raw foods for the summer months.

The ancient Chinese understood that with the cyclical movement of the sun throughout the four seasons there was literally more energy available in the summer than in the winter. In primitive societies it is easy to live according to these simple laws of nature; when it is dark, you can no longer work. But we have electric light and central-heating systems and tend to think that the whole year is much the same. The second chapter of *The Yellow Emperor's Classic of Internal Medicine* teaches us to live according to the four seasons, and in the winter we are told to rise later and to go to bed early, to keep ourselves to ourselves, and not to expend too much energy with external affairs. It's a kind of hibernation, a withdrawal of the self from the outside world; a time of contemplation, of reassessment and a gathering of strength. In this way we protect the energy of the kidneys.

This simple advice is usually rejected in favour of complex treatments with acupuncture, herbs, supplements or drugs, which of course may all have their uses, but it is not until we are to take simple steps to help ourselves that true healing can begin. Learning to conserve our energy is the main treatment for kidney weakness in Chinese medicine.

Over-action of this inward movement may manifest in fear and timidity, with an inability to grasp life and get on with things. As we are able to build up the strength of the kidneys, to conserve and preserve our energies through the winter months, eventually we may be able to respond to the natural movement of the spring, beginning deep within the earth in the depths of winter and finally bursting forth with renewed energy and vitality. It is by facing our fears that we gain wisdom, and wisdom is the natural virtue of the kidneys. This is a practical know-how that enables us to live wisely, a deep-rooted wisdom that helps us to conserve our energies, to grow and adapt according to our natural life cycles.

EXERCISES FOR THE KIDNEYS

Massage and stretches to invigorate the kidneys and the kidney meridian

1. Standing with the feet parallel and shoulder-width apart, place the hands over the lower abdomen and take a few deep breaths. When the breath feels calm and regular, take a deep breath in and stretch up on tiptoes, the hands stretching high

above the head. Release and breathe out. Repeat a few times (Fig. 82).

2. Return to the standing position, hands over the abdomen. Breathe deeply until the breath is calm and regular. Take a deep breath in and with the out-breath let the body fall forward over the legs, allowing the hands to relax wherever they are comfortable. Breathe normally in this position, relaxing and releasing the waist and lower back, until returning to the upright position with an inhalation. Take a few breaths and repeat (Fig. 83).

Check that the feet are still parallel; breathe deeply with the hands over the lower abdomen for a minute or so.

3. Rub the hands vigorously together until they are warm, then place them over the kidneys. Repeat three times (Fig. 84). With the palms of the hands over the kidneys, rub gently but gradually apply more pressure until the whole area feels warm and tingling. If there is any discomfort, continue with the first method, holding the kidneys with the warm hands.

Making a loose fist with the hands, lightly pummel the muscles either side of the spine from the end of the ribcage to the pelvis. Be gentle. If it feels good, continue for a few minutes, if not keep on with the holding and gentle rubbing.

Keeping the hands over the kidneys, take a deep breath in and, breathing out, bend back, supporting the back and waist with the hands (Fig. 85). Breathe in as you straighten up, and with the next out-breath allow the body to fall forwards over the legs with a forced exhalation, the hands relaxing down to the floor (Fig. 86); breathe in as you return to the upright position. Co-ordinate these movements with the breath, each time stretching with the exhalation, returning to the upright position with the inhalation.

Once you have co-ordinated the body movements with the rhythm of the breath co-ordinate the hand movements with the forward bend: moving the hands from the kidneys over the buttocks and down the backs of the legs to assist the flow of energy in the kidney and bladder meridians.

This short routine of exercises strengthens the kidneys, keeps flexibility in the lower back and invigorates the kidney and bladder meridians.

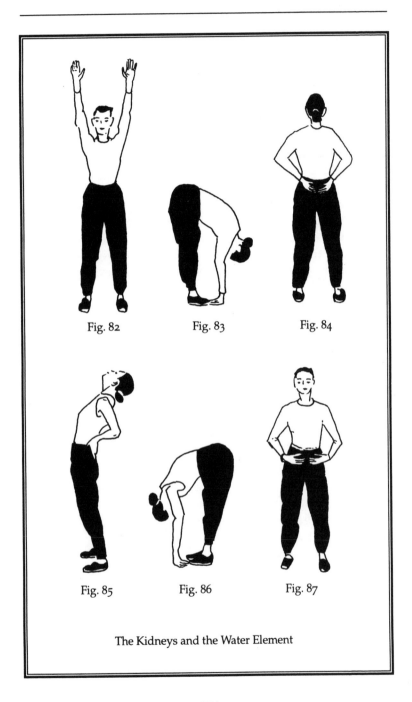

Fig. 82   Fig. 83   Fig. 84

Fig. 85   Fig. 86   Fig. 87

The Kidneys and the Water Element

Qi gong meditation

Assume the basic standing qi gong position, with the feet parallel, the knees slightly bent, the lower back straight and the tail-bone tucked in. Place the hands on the lower abdomen, covering the acupuncture points sea of qi (Ren 6) and gate to the origin (Ren 4, Plate 5). Focus the mind on the part of the abdomen covered by the hands. Breathe deeply and evenly, feeling the breath penetrating into the lower abdomen.

When you are able to feel the breath in the lower abdomen, allow the hands to move away from the body by gently lifting the forearms to form a circle – the fingertips facing each other and the palms facing towards the abdomen. You may feel a tingling in the fingertips or palms. This is your natural healing energy. Still focusing on the lower abdomen, feel the energy from the palm directed back into the abdomen, forming a circuit. Breathe naturally and close the eyes. Hold this position for five minutes (Fig. 87).

If the arms begin to ache, try to relax and release tension in the shoulders, but bring the hands back to the abdomen to rest if the arms or shoulders become too painful.

Open your eyes and bring the hands slowly to the lower abdomen, gathering in the qi and vitality to this lower centre. Stand quietly for a few moments.

Shake the hands, arms and shoulders, the feet, legs and hips. Jump lightly on the spot, releasing any tension the body has acquired in holding the position.

Standing upright with the feet together, stretch on to tiptoes, take a few breaths, then come quickly down on to the heels, jolting the legs and lower back. This ancient exercise has been practised for hundreds of years to strengthen the inner organs, massage the kidneys and stimulate the kidney and bladder meridians. Repeat a few times.

Sitting exercises for the kidney and bladder meridians

Sit on a mat with the legs stretched out in front of you. Move the body forward and the legs backwards so that the weight is on the tops of the thighs rather than the buttocks. Bend forward, holding with the hands around the feet, ankles or legs, whatever is comfortable. Keep the head up, so that the back is stretched and not hunched. With each out-breath try to move forward, releasing the stretch at the back of the knee (Fig. 88).

Both the kidney and bladder meridians have vital points at the back of the knees, and as at all joints, energy can easily stagnate here. It is at the knees that the more superficial flow of the meridian becomes deeper, and both the kidney and bladder meridians have a direct connection with their associated organs from these points at the knees. If the knees feel very stiff and tight, use the hands to massage the back of the knees, helping the muscles to release and relax as you stretch.

Holding the left foot with the right hand, bring it to rest on the right thigh, massaging the ball of the foot with the thumbs of both hands. On the point Kidney 1, gushing spring (Fig. 89), use gentle rotating movements with the right thumb, gradually moving to the inside edge of the foot (Kidney 2) and to the inner ankle bone. The kidney meridian turns around the inner ankle bone, and four of its major points lie in this small circle. Massage these points with gentle rotations, avoiding any jabbing or dragging movements. Repeat with the right foot.

If you can comfortably hold the ankles, reach forward with the hands and place the thumb gently over Kidney 6 and the forefinger over Bladder 62 (Plate 8). Rest in this position, supporting the head with a pillow on the legs or resting the forehead on a block (Fig. 90). If you cannot reach the ankles with the hands, rest the forehead on a chair and hold the backs of the knees. While stretching and invigorating the kidney and bladder channels, this position calms the mind and stimulates the yin and yang qiao mai, creating balance and harmony between yin and yang in the whole organism.

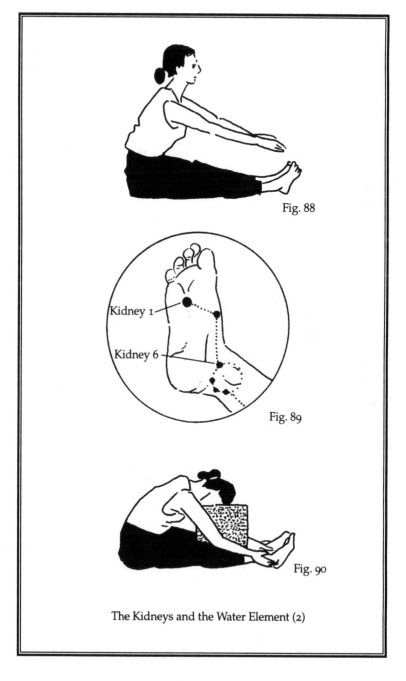

Fig. 88

Kidney 1

Kidney 6

Fig. 89

Fig. 90

The Kidneys and the Water Element (2)

THE WOOD ELEMENT AND THE LIVER

Wood is associated with spring, with expansion and growth. It is yang in nature and relates to the climate wind and to movement. Problems with the wood energy and with the liver tend to be of an excess nature, and the symptoms may be violent, whether manifesting as headaches, digestive problems or premenstrual symptoms. But as with each of the elements and their associated organs, as much damage may be caused by insufficiency as by excess and, clinically, many liver problems manifest as a result of repression and stagnation. Problems with the energetic field of the liver are generally helped by movement, and it is in this area that exercise can be most useful; whether it is by walking part of the way to work or taking up a serious physical disicipline, it is important to shake up the system, get rid of blockages and get the energy flowing freely.

All movement and exercise is beneficial, but competitive sports tend to emphasise one part of the body over the other, whereas disciplines such as yoga, tai ji and most martial arts are specially designed to work on the muscles of the whole body as well as on the subtle energy channels. They also work with the breath and concentration which is most important when aiming to bring about inner transformation.

Our bodies are all different, and we need the kind of movement and exercise that suits us. Hatha yoga stretches the muscles and aligns the body; tai ji is more fluid and gentle. A patient who suffered from severe liver symptoms, which manifested in outbursts of anger and migraine headaches, told me that he would often use a punch bag, which seemed to help restore his equilibrium. A popular qi gong exercise for the liver uses similar rhythmic punching movements, and when he learnt this exercise and how to co-ordinate his movement with the breath, it became a valuable tool in his recovery.

Physical exercise can help to overcome blockage in the body but it can also bring release to the mind. If we are feeling depressed and stuck, physical movement can begin to bring about energetic change which will eventually help us to move on in our lives, to change our minds and alter our perspective.

The liver in its relationship to the hun, or soul, flourishes with creative expression; the lack of creative expression can cause much of the anger and frustration associated with liver problems. Generations of women have thrown themselves into scrubbing and cleaning to cope with internal feelings of repression and anger, or simply as a way to release their energy. Just imagine the power if these feelings could be harnessed into creative expression!

Living in Japan after 5 years of art school training taught me that to be artistic or creative does not necessarily mean to paint or make pots, to write or to act, but that each action can become an act of creativity. In the same way that concentration on the breath and the intent can change a simple movement to a dynamic one, bringing the soul into our actions can change the mundane into the artistic. It is well illustrated in the Zen literature that each everyday task can be made into an art form, but I'm not advocating here that we just do the washing-up with extra concentration and awareness and transform it into an act of creativity, though I'm sure it is possible to do so. What is needed to help the healthy expansion of the liver energy is self-expression.

The hun is the personal soul, that individual part of you that seeks higher expression; it is your imagination and vision. What is important is that it is your own personal expression, and we all need to fulfil this in different ways. In the West we tend to create artistic hierarchies, where the fine arts are somewhere at the top of the list and needlework or gardening don't really figure. In Japan there is an equal appreciation of all artistic endeavour; whether it is 'artistic' depends on whether it captures the soul.

The important thing is to find what is right for you. In terms of your liver energy it is often doing the thing that you have always wanted to do. Don't aim so high that you immediately make it impossible, but think of small ways in which you can begin to give yourself some time and space for your own creativity. Join a creative writing class, a dance class; make time to work in the garden, or plan some interesting walks. Anything, so long as you give just a bit of time to yourself and your inner needs. Your soul is your responsibility.

Many of us are psychic in one way or another and our liver energy can also be repressed when we do not listen to our dreams and visions. This is just another aspect of our creativity, and if we refuse to listen, we can again cause blockage in the natural freeflow of the liver energy, causing headaches, often severe migraines, digestive problems, and possibly sexual problems. We all dream dreams, have hunches, occasionally have premonitions. These are often subtle feelings, and the more you listen, the more you will hear. Just take note. That's all that is necessary. Write down vivid dreams. Record your hunches, and maybe we will soon begin to realise that these gifts are not weird and abnormal but just a part of the vast creative capacity of our minds.

RELATING

The energy of wood and of spring is to move outwards. And as the fire element and the heart keep us in touch with heaven and our spirit, and the water element and the kidneys keep us in touch with the earth and the roots of our individuality, so the movement of wood and the liver keeps us in touch with humanity. The virtue associated with the liver is humanity and benevolence, the ability of mankind to reach out to others, and to treat others with kindness and compassion. And as the root of many wood problems lies in the lack of water, so many of the problems of human relationship are based on fear.

As the human spirit moves out in love it is often met with rejection and sometimes with violence. This can be devastating and a cause of real pain and suffering. Eventually we may decide that it is easier not to reach out at all, or to reach out only with a superficial part of ourselves while keeping our true feelings locked safely away.

It is not always possible for us to change our circumstances, but that does not mean that we cannot try to release negative emotions. Eastern medicine suggests that it is not necessary to understand and identify emotional patterns before they can be changed; in fact it is often impossible to understand our emotions until we are some distance away from them. Our rational minds want to identify and understand before we are ready to release our old patterns of behaviour, old wounds and scars that are in the way of our progress and are possibly having a detrimental effect on our health.

During an early acupuncture session in Japan, when I could speak very little of the language, and was with a practitioner who rarely spoke to his patients, I can remember crying for a full hour after one treatment, with a deep sadness that seemed as if it could have gone on for ever. I didn't know what it was about, and not a word was spoken, but I was given a safe, quiet place to be alone with my sorrow, and someone checked on me now and then and brought me tea. There seemed to be no need to understand the suffering, just an acceptance of it, and the space and time to let it go.

When I described the session later to my teacher he nodded in understanding, then added that many Westerners practising Eastern disciplines insist on employing the rational mind throughout their training. This has its value, but can lead to problems and in severe cases to insanity, as the mind comes across things that it cannot understand. We tend to overvalue our ability to understand with the rational mind, and forget that it does have its limitations. Sometimes it is necessary to suspend logic, to let go of the analytical mind.

It is always hard to look at something objectively if you're in the middle of it, even more so if you are trying to look at your emotions. So we may need to let go of our anger and frustration without a complete resolution of the surrounding situation. If energy can be balanced, whether with acupuncture, herbs, exercise or meditation, then in the new balanced state the situation may be reassessed and understood. Healing blockages in the liver energy and restoring freeflow can help us to heal our relationships. Healing our relationships can help the energies of the liver.

Learning to release our anger frees up the imagination and creative power, and by expressing our creativity we can begin to release our repressed anger.

EXERCISES FOR THE LIVER

Side stretches

Standing straight with the feet parallel and shoulder-width apart, and with the hands by the sides, take a few deep breaths. Take a deep breath in and on the out-breath stretch the right hand down the leg as far as you can, taking care not to move the body forwards but remaining in the same vertical plane. (Imagine that you are standing between two panes of glass and must move to the side without touching them.) Breathe in as you return to the upright position. Repeat to the left (Fig. 91).

Consciously relax and release the side that is stretching, particularly the side ribs and the neck. Complete five stretches to each side.

To increase the stretch, repeat the movement with the right hand stretching down the leg and the left hand over the head. Breathe in as you stretch the left hand straight up beside the ear, breathe out as you stretch to the side. Remain in the position for a few breaths, breathing naturally. Repeat on the opposite side (Fig. 92).

Body swings

Preparation:
Stand in the basic qi gong position, feet parallel and hip-width apart. Allow the knees to bend naturally, checking that the hips are level.

Bring the hands to the lower abdomen and stand for a few moments breathing deeply. Feel that the feet are strongly connected to the ground, the kidney meridian providing the root that goes deep into the earth. Feel that the feet are evenly balanced, with equal weight on the heels and the ball of the foot, on the outside and inside edges. The legs should feel strong and firm.

Movement:
Bringing the hands away from the abdomen to hang loosely at the sides, move the shoulders to the left, looking over the left shoulder, and then to the right, looking over the right shoulder; let this movement develop into a rhythmic swing, the arms and chest feeling light and free, the lower body stable. Keep the hips parallel and facing forwards as much as you can as this ensures the stretch is strongest around the side waist and lower ribcage, which contain vital points on the liver and gall-bladder meridians, as well as stimulating the internal organs (Fig. 93).

This simple motion invigorates the gall-bladder and liver meridians and ensures freeflow in the area of the abdomen.

Invigorating qi gong

Standing in the basic qi gong position, with the feel parallel and the knees slightly bent, bring the hands into loose fists and hold them, facing upwards, at either side of the waist.

Take a deep breath in, exhale through the mouth with a loud 'haaa!' as you punch the right hand straight forwards, turning the fist as you do so.

Inhale as you draw the fist back to its original position at the waist, and exhale through the mouth with a loud 'haa!' as you punch with the left hand. Keep the feet and hips strong and move them as little as possible (Fig. 94).

Repeat with a good strong rhythm, getting faster as you go. When you get the rhythm right you begin to sound like a steam train building up speed. Gradually decrease speed and take a few deep breaths before beginning another cycle.

If you feel breathless or dizzy at any time, stop immediately

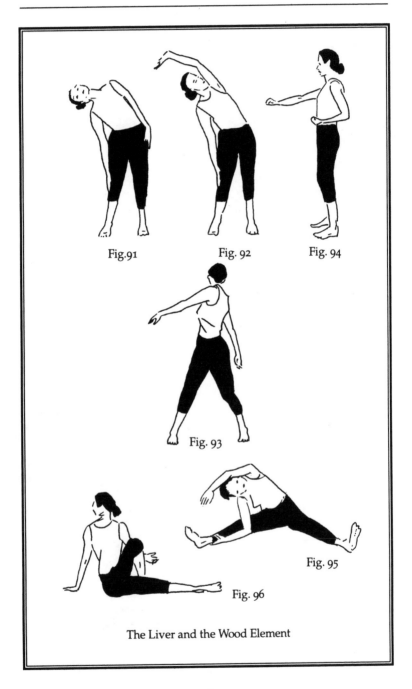

Fig. 91

Fig. 92

Fig. 94

Fig. 93

Fig. 95

Fig. 96

The Liver and the Wood Element

and take deep breaths. Bend forward from the waist, and let the upper body completely relax.

Exercises that work specifically to invigorate the liver in this way can stimulate the release of toxins; if you begin to feel nausea or develop a headache, this is often a sign of toxin release. Work with the more gentle exercises for a few weeks before attempting the more stimlating exercises. If you do suffer from headaches or nausea after performing these exercises, drink plenty of water to make sure that the released toxins are eliminated.

Liver and gall-bladder meridian stretches

Sitting on a mat, arrange the weight so that you are sitting forward with the lower spine as straight as possible. Move the legs as far apart as they will go without strain.

Sit upright with the spine straight; stretch the right arm along the right leg. Breathe in as you take the left arm over the left ear, and, breathing out, bring the body sideways towards the right leg. Take a few breaths, relaxing into the stretch as you breathe out (Fig. 95). Repeat to the left.

If you have not done much exercise recently you may feel very stiff in this position. Be gentle, as the inner thigh muscles are delicate and can easily be strained. Don't worry if you cannot stretch very far – the meridians will still get the benefit of the stretch, and the muscles will gradually loosen. In Chinese medical theory, the liver governs the muscles, and if there is a lack of freeflow, or a lack of nourishment to the muscles, these movements can be very helpful. Relax into the position, never forcing, but allowing the weight of the upper body to stretch the sides and the hips gently. The gall-bladder meridian flows along the side of the body, and has two points (Gall-bladder 22 and 23) at the side of the breast which are often used by acupuncturists for breast problems. This exercise provides this little stimulated area with a wonderful stretch that helps the circulation through the breasts. The breast symptoms that often accompany PMT can also be helped by this meridian stretch. Many premenstrual symptoms involve the lack of freeflow in the liver and gall-bladder meridians, and these exercises can be particularly helpful.

Spinal twist

Sitting with the spine straight and the legs stretched fowards, place the right foot on the floor beside the left knee, the right knee pointing upwards. Take in a deep breath. With the exhalation twist to the left, placing the right arm inside the right knee, the hand on the outer left calf. Place the left hand behind your back and look over your left shoulder. The inside of the right knee should press against the outside of the right arm to help the body twist towards the left. Breathe naturally. Repeat by bringing up the left knee and twisting to the right (Fig. 96).

The eyes:
It is important in many of these liver exercises to use the eyes. In traditional qi gong texts the instructions are to 'stare angrily'. The eyes are the orifice connected to the liver and these details ensure that the whole complex of the liver is invigorated by the exercise.

Walking

Walking is one of the most natural ways to aid the freeflow of energy in the body and therefore to aid the function of the liver. All walking is beneficial – but if you can walk where there are trees and are able simultaneously to enjoy natural surroundings, so much the better. The wood element craves expansion, open spaces, fresh air. It loves the beauty of nature, and walking is particularly beneficial in the springtime, when energies are naturally expanding and you can literally inhale the new vibrancy in the air.

If you are aiming to walk for exercise, try not to carry much with you. A small rucksack is indispensable for allowing the arms to be free. Bags carried on the shoulder tend to create imbalance in the posture, and do not free up the arms. Be aware of your breath, and try to breathe deeply and evenly. At some time walk quite fast with the arms swinging. This creates a similarly invigorating effect as much of the standing qi gong. As with all exercise, if you walk consciously, with attention to the breath, you increase the therapeutic effect.

THE METAL ELEMENT AND THE LUNGS

The lungs relate to the metal element, to autumn, and to the movement of condensation. The lungs govern the qi or the breath and respond to breathing exercises of many kinds. All exercise works on the lungs, and if the lungs are strong and healthy strenuous exercise can stimulate and invigorate both the heart and the lungs. But if the lungs are weak, it is important not to exhaust the energy, and Oriental exercise tends to stress calm, controlled movement and breathing, rather than panting and getting out of breath. This is not seen as necessary to exercise the heart and lungs.

If the lungs are weak they need to be coaxed gradually back into activity by slowly increasing the duration – both of each individual breath and the time spent in breathing exercises. In most lung problems the lung capacity is diminished, and especially with asthma the muscles in the upper back and intercostals tend to be tight. If you work too hard, too quickly, the muscles may relax for a while but often seize up the following day. Qi gong exercises specifically developed for the lungs gradually enhance the capacity of the lungs, bringing back the elasticity of the muscles, while simultaneously stimulating the lung meridian and its major acupuncture points.

The first point of the lung meridian is at the side of the chest in the groove made by the shoulder joint. If you hunch the shoulders forward or move them up towards the ears, this area is immediately compressed, and the flow of the lung meridian is impeded. The same movement creates tension in the upper back, affecting the back lung points and the nerve supply to the lungs. In this way posture and lung weakness become a vicious circle, each damaging the other in a downward spiral: weakness in the chest creates the compensatory and protective movement of hunching the shoulders; this movement in turn weakens the lungs even more by interrupting both nerve and energy supplies.

Grief and sadness, the emotions associated with the lungs, also create this protective movement, which is well illustrated in the Chinese character for sadness and oppression, which shows a hand pressing down on the heart. It is a movement in resonance with the autumn and the contraction of metal. Many people experience lung problems after a time of deep sadness or loss, and the lack of joy, which we discussed in relation to the heart, also affects the lungs. Both the heart and lungs work in the upper heater to give the body its natural rhythms.

This kind of oppression in the chest from sadness or lack of joy makes the breath shallow, as we breathe from just a small area at the top of the lungs. According to the Chinese view of energy production, the air that we breathe is the essential last step in providing the energy that we use every day. If our breathing is too shallow, our available energy is diminished.

Shallow breathing can be seen as a way of not fully participating in life. It is an avoidance of fully committing ourselves, holding something back, not totally engaging in reality. Maybe we are in a situation that we know is not right for us, but rather than confront it we just live on the edge of our life – not fully present. Deep breathing is a way of embracing life, of embracing the present and of embracing yourself.

A patient with severe energy depletion, diagnosed by her GP as having Chronic Fatigue Syndrome, had had various alternative treatments which had kept her stable but she was still unable to return to work. Sometimes she would appear completely normal, her spirit was good, her voice strong and clear, and it was not until I saw her on one of her bad days that I noticed that her breathing was completely erratic. In traditional Chinese pulse diagnosis the doctor will often compare the beats of the pulse to the breathing, and while watching her breathe I saw it had lost all rhythm; sometimes she would almost forget to breathe.

As we saw in Part 1 (p. 52), the po, or bodily soul, relates to the lungs and governs the autonomic nervous system, giving rhythm and co-ordination to the deep function of the body, which we assume to be out of conscious control. Yoga theory teaches us that by controlling the breath we can eventually control those deep inner functions, such as the beating of the heart, the contraction and expansions of the digestive system, the opening and closing of the pores.

That these functions can be controlled by the breath suggests that if the breath is erratic, these functions may also become erratic, disturbing such deep bodily rhythms as the workings of the bowels and digestive system, sleeping patterns, and even causing an erratic heart beat.

Introducing breathing exercises which she could do even in bed – simply counting the breaths to ten and beginning again – began the slow journey towards full recovery. After a week or so, she began to count to four with each inhalation and exhalation, gradually making them longer and deeper, until she was finally able to practise standing qi gong. As soon as she felt strong enough she began a regular swimming routine. Swimming, especially backstroke, is a wonderful way to exercise the lungs, and with the weight of the body supported by the water, the lungs are free to open and expand. As long as the concentration is focused on the breath, swimming or walking can be just as effective as qi gong, and many people enjoy the extra activity to keep them motivated. It is the rhythm that is important – the rhythm of the breath, the rhythm of the movement and the regularity of the practice.

EXERCISES TO STRENGTHEN THE LUNGS

Breathing exercises

These breathing exercises can be performed sitting or lying down. If you prefer to lie down, or are unable to sit for extended periods, lie flat and place a small pillow or rolled-up towel between the shoulder blades, which helps the chest to open and the shoulder blades to move back and down. Open the armpits and rotate the arms so that the palms face comfortably upwards. This ensures that the circulation in the lung meridian is unhampered. If the back aches, draw up the knees (Fig. 97).

If sitting, sit comfortably with the back straight and focus the mind on the breath. Make sure that the armpits are slightly open and that the arms are not too close to the sides of the body. Feel that the chest has plenty of space to expand sideways, and that air can circulate freely. Placing the hands with the palms upwards on the knees or in the lap naturally brings the arms into the correct position. Relax the shoulders (Fig. 98).

Feel the air as it moves gently through the nostrils, the gentle expansion and contraction of the ribcage. Concentrating the mind completely on the breath, begin counting slowly to four with each inhalation, and to four with each exhalation. The count should be slow, and if you struggle to reach four, begin with a count of three. Repeat for five minutes.

Gradually increased the count of the out-breath. Begin by breathing in to a count of four, and out to a count of six. Then increase to eight, ten and twelve. This is most effective if increased gradually over a few weeks until you feel completely comfortable with the extended out-breath.

If you have breathing difficulties you should not attempt to lengthen the breath until the count to four feels totally natural. If at any time during the practice you feel out of breath, stop and take a few deep breaths before continuing.

Qi gong to strengthen the lungs

Assume the basic qi gong standing position, with the feet parallel and hip-width apart and the knees relaxed. Raise the hands to chest height, palms facing the floor, keeping the elbows relaxed and slightly bent. As if you are picking up a delicate object, bring the tip of the thumb and the tip of the first finger together. This hand movement or mudra connects the lung and large intestine meridians and is maintained throughout the exercise (Fig. 99).

With an inhalation, move the hands apart until your arms describe part of a large circle – not totally extended, but wide enough to give a stretch to the chest; push outwards with the inside of the wrists (Fig. 100). Hold the breath while turning the hands and arms, so that the palms face upwards. Exhale while bringing the hands together (Fig. 101). Turn the hands as you begin to inhale for the next cycle.

This arm movement helps the natural expansion and contraction of the lungs, stimulates the lung meridian and the vital lung meridian acupoints around the wrist.

Breathe slowly and deeply, keeping the shoulders relaxed. Continue for five minutes, resting to relax the shoulders if they become too painful. Try to relax the muscles in the arms and shoulders as you work; if you can work through the pain, it is always better than stopping. If you stop, try to keep the rhythm of the breath. Gradually increase the exercise time to ten minutes.

Lung and large intestine meridian stretch

Standing straight with the feet parallel and slightly wider than shoulder-width apart, rotate the shoulders first one way then the other as described in the general warm-up section (p. 127). Pull the shoulders up towards the ears and then let them relax. Repeat a few times.

Take the hands behind the back and link the thumbs, pulling the hands away from each other. Maintaining this hand position, take a deep breath in and, breathing out, bend forwards, stretching the hands upwards and backwards. Relax, and repeat (Fig. 102).

If we want to help our lungs we must breathe. The more stressed and busy we are, the more shallow our breathing tends to become and our shoulders become tense and hunched forward. Wherever we are, whatever we are doing, it is important to stop for a few minutes now and again and think about the breath. Am I breathing regularly? Am I

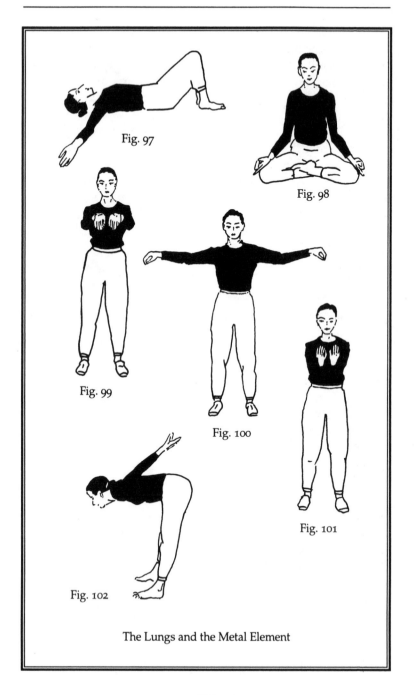

Fig. 97

Fig. 98

Fig. 99

Fig. 100

Fig. 101

Fig. 102

The Lungs and the Metal Element

breathing deeply? Am I breathing at all? In times of severe stress and tension, whether in emotional crisis or extreme stress at work, we often forget to breathe, holding the breath for extended periods, or breathing very shallowly from the top of the lungs. Just stop, take a few minutes, and breathe deeply. The lungs are the 'master of qi' and therefore master the available energy in the organism. The Chinese word qi can be translated as both breath and energy. Our breath is our energy, our energy is our breath. Strengthen the breath and you strengthen the energy.

THE EARTH ELEMENT AND THE SPLEEN

The spleen relates to the centre, and to the element earth. Its movement is to circulate and distribute. It governs transformation and transportation. In the seasons it relates to later summer, the time of harvests when the earth element facilitates the difficult change from the expansion of summer to the contraction of autumn. If our earth energy is low, this change may be particularly difficult. But, in the traditional Chinese calendar, the earth element also relates to the two-week period between each season. The earth thus regulates all change, and the other four elements relate harmoniously to each other through the earth: the earth balances the fire and the water, the wood and the metal in their oppositions, creating change and flow.

Within the physical body the spleen and its earth element partner, the stomach, govern the assimilation of food, the stomach taking in and processing the more physical aspects of food, the spleen the more energetic. We saw in Part 1 how the spleen governs the five tastes and is said to be responsible for the distribution of the more subtle aspects of nutrition to the individual organs. The taste of a particular food is its energetic signature; it shows us what the food will do within the body. The sour taste of a lemon contracts, and it is this movement of contraction that allows the springing up of the liver energy. Too much contraction and the springing-up movement cannot occur. The bitter taste stimulates the heart by a kind of quickening. If the heart energy is weak this may cause palpitations, as we have all experienced from that cup of coffee too many. The five tastes must be balanced, and one way to judge a good Oriental meal is in its balance of the five tastes. The Japanese use five flavourings in most of their food: sugar, vinegar, salt, soy and miso (fermented soy bean curd) which, if used in harmony, create a balance of taste. It is traditional, however, to create these five tastes with natural foodstuffs rather than condiments. Vegetables and grains are said to be sweet and from the earth; seaweeds are salty and from the water; bitter tastes are generally roasted on a fire; sour tastes from the wood, and foods are combined accordingly. In China, many hospitals of traditional Chinese medicine have a restaurant attached, where your food prescription can be fulfilled.

In the West diet is altogether a different matter. When a centre for alternative medicine was established in the chronic pain department of a hospital in Boston, practitioners of all disciplines were invited to take part in this exciting trial of alternative medicine. The project went ahead and was successful in all but one area – diet. Each practitioner had his or her own opinions on diet – opinions that varied widely and were often totally contradictory. Many patients would be given advice by one practitioner one day and conflicting advice by another the next. For example, Chinese medicine advises eating only cooked food, suggesting that raw foods create cold and damp in the spleen which can lead to the excess production of mucus. This is a sharp contradiction to the many raw food diets advocated in the West.

More than any other aspect of health, diet is an individual thing. Some of us have a fast metabolism and need to be slowed down by carbohydrates; others have a slow metabolism which tends to get glued up with too much stodgy food. We need to find out what is good for us individually, and to get back to a few simple basic rules, such as warming the cold, cooling the heat, invigorating the sluggish and calming the over-active. But according to Chinese medicine often it is not what we eat that is at the root of the problem but rather the way that we eat and our ability to absorb and transform. Instead of discussing which foods to eat, the Chinese medical practitioner first aims to balance the spleen energy, for unless the spleen is able to absorb nutrients and transform them into useable form within the body, no amount of dietary advice will solve the problem. Unless the body is assimilating properly, however many supplements we take they may not be effective.

The obsession that tends to accompany many diets can compound the problems of an already weakened spleen energy. Obsession is the negative emotion related to the spleen, and overthinking or obsessional thought can create a spiral of energy that knots and obstructs, so that we either feel bloated and lack appetite or continually crave to be full. Most addictions or obsessions indicate a weakness in the associated organ, and as smoking addictions may be masking an inherent weakness in the lungs, eating disorders of all kinds are generally related to imbalance in the spleen energy.

People of all shapes and sizes suffer from spleen weakness. Whether the problem is obesity or the inability to put on weight, the answer is very often simply to strengthen the spleen; according to our constitutional type, the spleen weakness will manifest in different ways.

The relationship of the liver to the spleen is another interesting aspect of digestive problems. In the five-element cycle the liver is said to have a controlling effect on the spleen, and those of us who lose weight easily will often have a strong liver energy, which is exerting too strong an influence on the spleen. This kind of over-activity of the liver may manifest in a wiry, muscular body, over-active, being always on the go. Once the spleen is weakened in this way, the problem is compounded as the spleen is unable to check the over-aggressive activity of the liver. This is a typical excess yang symptom, and needs to be countered with yin activities: eat regularly, rest after meals. If you exercise, concentrate on the slower, more relaxing exercises. Your body needs calm and regularity.

If you tend to put on weight easily, the liver energy may be blocked and unable to activate the spleen. You may tend to migraines when the frustrated liver energy suddenly breaks through, which happens especially around the time of menstruation. The Chinese medical classics say that '... anger triumphs over obsessive thought', and in the same way that the expansive energy of the liver can stimulate the spleen into action in the emotional realm, so it can do the same in the physical. If your spleen is sluggish and you tend to gain weight easily, activating the liver energy with exercise, and paying attention to your own creative expression may be the best way to move forward.

MOXA, MASSAGE AND EXERCISE

Moxibustion:
The spleen likes to be warm and dry and responds very well to treatment with moxibustion. 'Moxa' is a herb (artemisa vulgaris) which is used by Chinese medical practitioners in conjunction with, or often instead of, acupuncture. In my clinical practice I often suggest that my clients use moxa for simple treatments at home – and especially to strengthen the spleen and stomach.

Moxa can be used in cigar-like rolls to warm and strengthen the energy in a particular area, and in small adhesive cones for more direct stimulation of a specific acupuncture point. Moxa sticks and cones can be obtained from acupuncture and Chinese herbal suppliers and some of the larger clinics of Chinese medicine. Two specific points, Stomach 36 and Spleen 6 (Fig. 103), are widely used in conjunction for general strengthening of the spleen and the earth element. Twice-weekly treatment with stick-on moxa cones or with a moxa stick will be very effective in strengthening the spleen and stomach (Fig. 104).

When locating the acupuncture point for this kind of treatment, run the finger gently over the skin in the area illustrated. You will often feel a depression or a spot where the skin is more sensitive to the touch. Both of these points have quite a large area of influence, so accuracy is not so vital as with other more precise locations.

If using stick-on moxa cones, burn three cones on the point

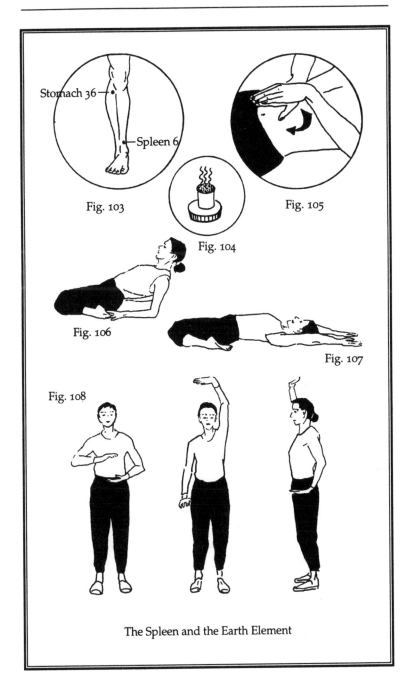

Stomach 36

Spleen 6

Fig. 103

Fig. 104

Fig. 105

Fig. 106

Fig. 107

Fig. 108

The Spleen and the Earth Element

for one treatment. Allow the cone to burn down until it is too hot to bear. Have an ashtray handy for the used cones. Light the cones in sequence so that two cones do not become hot at the same time. Use both points on both legs for the most effective treatment.

If using a moxa stick, move the lighted stick in small circles around the point, about an inch or so from the body. When the area becomes hot, move on to the next point, rotating the four points in this way for ten minutes or so.

ABDOMINAL MASSAGE

Lying comfortably on the floor, rest the two hands over the navel, the right hand over the left. Breathe gently and evenly. With slight pressure from the right hand over the left, which remains completely relaxed, begin to make circular movements around the navel in a clockwise direction. Gradually make the circles larger until you reach the ribcage. Begin again. Repeat this three times (Fig. 105).

This gentle massage aids digestion and relieves tension in the abdomen. It is especially useful in constipation.

SPLEEN AND STOMACH MERIDIAN STRETCHES

Sit between the feet with soles of the feet upwards, toes pointing back. If this position is very easy for you, move the weight on to the elbows (Fig. 106) and lie with the back stretched along the floor. For added stretch move the arms above the head and relax them on the floor (Fig. 107). This is a wonderfully relaxing stretch which invigorates the spleen and stomach meridians and tones the internal organs. It is one of the few exercises that can be performed after eating, as it aids digestion.

If you cannot sit comfortably between the feet, use a firm cushion or pad to raise the buttocks until the knees are comfortable. Arrange cushions or pillows so that you are able to relax back, making sure that the spine is straight and the

Table 5: Five Element Therapy

	Fire	Water	Wood	Metal	Earth
Organ:	Heart	Kidneys	Liver	Lungs	Spleen
Movement:	Upward	Downward	Outward	Inward	Circular
Needs:	Calm	Warmth	Movement	Rhythm	Centredness
Body therapy:	Meditation	Rest	Exercise	Breathing	Diet
Soul therapy:	Regaining our rituals	Overcoming fears	Creative expression	Releasing the past	Staying centred

head well supported. There should be some stretch in the knees, but do not remain in the position if the knees are painful.

Once you are comfortable, this is a resting position and can be held for at least five minutes. If the knees ache, do a little every day until they loosen up. Some people find this position easy – for others it is one of the most difficult. But as with all these meridian stretches, it is not the final accomplished pose that is important but the stretch that you experience. It can be just as beneficial if performed with cushions and blocks.

QI GONG FOR BALANCING THE CENTRE

Standing in the basic qi gong position, imagine that you are holding a ball in front of the navel, the right hand under the left.

Breathe in, and on the out-breath stretch the right hand above the head, pushing upwards with the palm, and push the left hand down by the left side, palm facing the floor.

Breathe in as you bring the hands to cross in front of the navel, pushing the right hand down by the right side, and the left hand up over the head.

Repeat with a rhythmical movement, adjusting the breath to the movement, the movement to the breath. Imagine that the palm of one hand is connecting with heaven, while the other is connecting with the earth. This movement is called uniting heaven and earth, and is one of the most ancient exercises for the spleen and stomach (Fig. 108).

COMMON IMBALANCES

Practical Remedies for
Everyday Problems

In Part 5 we take a brief look at some common problems and begin to devise ways of approaching them through the Chinese system. We will look at the signs and symptoms, make a diagnosis and decide where to progress from there. By thinking about the problem we begin to bring clarity – not by worry or obsession, which leads nowhere, but by focusing our attention and asking ourselves a few basic questions. As always, the important thing is to look within, to listen to your body. Your body holds the answers.

HEADACHES

The symptoms associated with headaches generally indicate an excess of yang energy in the head. There may be many reasons for this and we will attempt to discuss a few of the most common patterns. In imbalance, yang energy tends to accumulate in the head, and this must be checked by balancing the yin and yang energies in the body.

IMBALANCE OF YIN AND YANG

Symptoms:
- Pain tends to be at the back of the head, or over the brow
- Head is hot
- Neck and shoulders tight

• Lower back or feet cold
• May wake with headache symptoms

Too much yang in the head tends to manifest with heat and throbbing pain; it may be a symptom of fever or simply the result of too much thinking or stress. In more severe cases of imbalance, the lower parts of the body may feel cold. If the muscles in the shoulders become tight the meridians flowing between the head and the body become restricted, and there is no longer an easy exchange of yin and yang. For this particular pattern we will be working with the bladder and kidney meridians, the du mai (Plate 4) and the yin and yang qiao mai (Plate 8) to regulate the yin and yang. These massage and stretching techniques are all covered in the section on stimulating the meridian system (pp. 119–40). Where new points are introduced I will explain more thoroughly.

• Massaging the sole of the foot and point Kidney 1
When there is an excess of energy in the head, there is generally a corresponding lack of energy in the lower body. One of the most safe and effective ways of treating headaches is to work on the feet.

Vigorously massage the sole of the foot with the thumbs (see above, Fig. 14), paying attention to the point Kidney 1. If the feet feel cold, it will help to soak them in warm water. Chronic problems of this kind can be alleviated if you soak the feet regularly in a ginger bath. Take a few slices of raw ginger root and boil them in a pan of water. Simmer for about half an hour. Add this to a bowl of cooler water and soak the feet for at least ten minutes. The ginger will warm the feet and invigorate the circulation in the meridians, drawing the excess energy away from the upper part of the body.

• Rubbing the kidneys
Rub the palms of the hands together until they feel hot. When the hands are hot, place them over the kidneys. Repeat three times. Rubbing the hands until they are hot, place them again over the kidneys and rub vigorously 20 times over the kidney area. Rest and repeat three times (Fig. 44).

● Stretching the neck
Sitting with the spine straight, take a deep breath in. With the out-breath, bring the chin slowly down to the chest, stretching the back of the neck. Breathe in as you return to the upright position. Breathe out as you slowly drop the head back, breathe in as you return to the upright. Repeat (Fig. 109).

It is important that these simple movements are performed slowly, with concentration and awareness. Fast or jerky movements could make the condition worse.

● Massaging point Bladder 10
Bring the hands to the back of the neck, fingers touching at the base of the skull. Move the fingers slowly away from the centre until they naturally fall into a depression either side of the central muscle. This is easy to feel if you bend the head slightly forward. Massage these points gently with the fingertips working over the muscles (Fig. 110).

● Soothing the forehead
Bring the hands to the forehead, the fingertips meeting at the centre between the brows. With a light pressure draw the fingers back to the side hairline.

● Massaging points Bladder 1 and Bladder 2
With the middle finger of both hands press either side of the bridge of the nose at the inner corner of the eye (Fig. 111). Raise the fingers to the inner end of the eyebrow and press. Try resting the elbows on a table and allowing the head to rest on the fingers.

● Releasing the brain
Sit on a mat with the legs stretched out in front of you. Move the body forward and the legs backwards so that the weight is on the tops of the thighs rather than the buttocks. Bend forward, resting the forehead on a chair. Use padding if necessary. Close your eyes and completely relax the head. The spine should feel a slight stretch and you should be aware of the weight of the head as it drops on to the support.

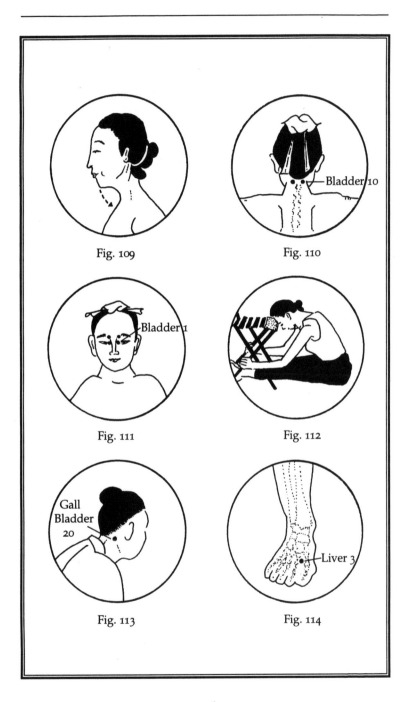

Fig. 109

Fig. 110

Fig. 111

Fig. 112

Fig. 113

Fig. 114

Be comfortable, adjusting the position until you can completely relax for ten minutes or so (Fig. 112).

● Walking to balance yin and yang qiao mai
With their main treatment points either side of the ankle bones, yin and yang qiao mai are invigorated and balanced simply by walking. Walking with a good regular stride in the open air can be one of the most effective cures for this kind of headache.

● Concentrating on the lower abdomen
When there is an excess of yang energy in the head, it is important to remove the concentration from the head and to bring the awareness into the lower abdomen. While you have a headache try not to use the eyes or the brain as this immediately activates the yang in the head. If this is not possible, punctuate periods of activity with times of rest. Close your eyes and move the attention to the lower abdomen as if you are withdrawing your sight from the outside world and looking within. Be gentle, do not force it as this immediately activates the brain and introduces tension. Imagine that you are breathing into the lower abdomen and if it helps you to concentrate, count the breaths from one to ten.

Long-term treatments:
● Circulation of light
Though the circulation of light meditation is not advised while you have a headache, it is possibly the most effective way to balance the yin and yang in the body in the long term.

● Balancing yin and yang qiao mai
Sit on a mat with the legs stretched out in front of you. Move the body forward and the legs backwards so that the weight is on the tops of the thighs rather than the buttocks. Bend forward. If you can comfortably hold the ankles, reach forward with the hands and place the thumb gently over Kidney 6 and the forefinger over Bladder 62 (Plate 8). Rest in this position, supporting the head with a pillow on the legs or

resting the forehead on a block or a chair (Fig. 90 and Fig. 112). If you cannot reach the ankles with the hands, rest the forehead on a chair and hold the backs of the knees. While stretching and invigorating the kidney and bladder channels, this position calms the mind and stimulates the yin and yang qiao mai, creating balance and harmony between yin and yang in the whole organism.

AGGRESSIVE LIVER ENERGY

- Symptoms tend to be at the side of the head, in one temple, or often affecting one eye
- Often violent, can be accompanied by nausea
- Visual disturbance
- Can be associated with feelings of anger, rage or frustration
- Likely to occur premenstrually

The liver energy has a naturally expansive movement; the liver meridian is the only yin meridian that has a deep pathway to the top of the head, and its yang wood-element partner, the gall-bladder meridian, covers the whole of the side of the head with its zigzag pathway. The gall-bladder meridian flows over the temples and penetrates the outer corner of the eye.

Wood-type headaches are often violent; the symptoms can come and go, and sometimes move from side to side. They are likely to cause visual disturbance as the eye is the associated orifice of the wood element. This could vary from blurred vision to the full-blown visual disorders experienced by some migraine sufferers.

Headaches caused by aggressive liver energy are often the most difficult to treat clinically: if they are chronic and do not respond to treatments to calm the liver, a deeper look into the long-term causes of the condition may be required; often there is an underlying frustration or suppressed anger. While working on a deeper level with emotional causes, it is always possible to restore the freeflow in the liver and gall-bladder meridians with the following simple actions.

● Rest the eyes:
The eyes are related to many different types of headaches, and closing the eyes immediately allows the head to relax. Rub the palms together until the hands are hot, and place the hands over the eyes. Repeat ten times (Fig. 30).

● Massage point Gall-bladder 20:
At the nape of the neck, in the depression an inch or so back from the ears is the important acupuncture point feng chi. Massaging this point allows the excess energy in the gall-bladder meridian to drain away from the head. Put your hands over your ears, and with your thumb, locate the depression at the side of the base of the skull. Massage gently with circular movements (Fig. 113).

● Stretching the neck:
When there is an excess of energy in the head, the neck often feels stiff and the shoulders tight. In the case of excess liver energy, it is most important to stretch the sides of the neck. Take a deep breath in, and with the out-breath bring the left ear towards the left shoulder, creating a stretch to the right side of the neck. Do not force, but allow the weight of the head to create the stretch. Take a few natural breaths while relaxing into the stretch. Repeat to the other side (Fig. 28).

● Massaging the shoulders:
Bring the right hand up to the left shoulder, supporting the right elbow in the left hand. With the pads of the three fingers press gently into the shoulders, moving from the neck towards the shoulder joint. In the centre of the top of the shoulder is the point Gall-bladder 21. This may be painful and should be massaged gently, with circular movements. This point helps the energy to move downwards in the body. Repeat to the other side (Fig. 26).

It is important to perform these movements on both sides of the body, even if the pain is one-sided, as it helps to balance left and right meridians. In the case of aggressive liver energy, shoulder massage should always be gentle. Though more force may feel good at the time, the muscles can overreact and go into spasm, compounding the problem.

● Massaging point Liver 3:
This is the most commonly used point (Fig. 114) for all liver disorders and it is very effective in calming excess liver yang. Massaging points on the feet is often the preferred treatment for headaches, drawing the excess energy down without fear of over-stimulating the head.

Long-term treatments:
All the exercises suggested for the liver and the wood element in Part 4 can be used when you do not have a headache, though walking and fresh air may also help to alleviate symptoms as well as working in the longer term.

ENERGY DEPLETION

Symptoms:
● Cold, tight feeling in the head
● Pain often at the top of the head
● Lower body cold
● Lower back aches
● Tiredness

Another common cause of headaches is energy depletion, which may be accompanied by a feeling of dizziness. The pain is often at the top of the head, but can be all over. The blood vessels in the head are generally constricted and the head feels tight. It is most important to rest and keep warm. The suggested treatments are to increase the energy and to warm the channels and meridians so that the circulation can flow again. Direct treatment on the head is not recommended.

● Moxa to Ren 4 and 6
Lie back comfortably propped up on pillows. You should be able to see and touch your lower abdomen without moving. Using a moxa stick (Fig. 115), warm the two points gate to the

origin and sea of qi (Ren 4 and 6, Fig. 116). Used together these two points stimulate the energy of the whole body.

● Massage to kidneys
Rub the hands together until they are warm. Place them at the back of the waist over the kidneys (Fig. 44). Repeat three times. Gently rub the kidney area from the bottom of the lower ribs to the top of the pelvis. If possible, get someone to do it for you!

● Moxa to Kidney 3, Stomach 36
Use stick-on moxa cones on the points Kidney 3 at the inner ankle (Fig. 117) and Stomach 36 just below the knee (Fig. 118). These two points have a deep strengthening action similar to that of Ren 4 and 6, but also act to stimulate the flow of energy in the meridians.

EYE STRAIN

Many headaches are related to eye strain and exercises can be very helpful, especially if you incorporate them in a regular preventive programme. Palming the eyes by rubbing the palms briskly together and placing the warm palms over the eyes can be done at any time and is particularly useful if you are working at a computer screen. This simple exercise is recommended in all traditions of healing in the East. If you spend much of your day doing close work, remember to rest your eyes at regular intervals. Look out of the window, preferably at distant green objects or the sky.

● Palming
Sitting in a relaxed position with the spine straight, rub the hands together vigorously until they are hot. Place the hands over the eyes, the centre of the palm over the centre of the eyeball. If you are at a desk, rest your elbows on the desk and allow your head to rest in the palms (Fig. 119). Relax the head and neck. Remain still for two to three minutes with the eyes closed. Repeat three times.

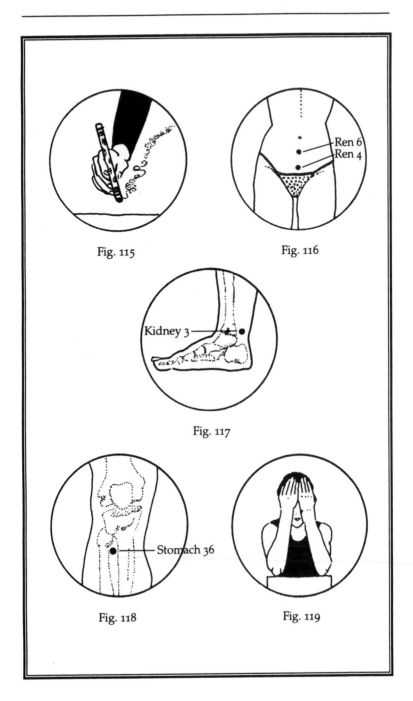

Fig. 115

Fig. 116

Fig. 117

Fig. 118

Fig. 119

● Stimulating the meridians

With the thumb and forefinger, pinch along the eyebrows, from the centre outwards, stimulating the points on the bladder, gall-bladder and triple-heater meridians. These points all help to revitalise the eyes and also stimulate the meridian function (Fig. 31).

● Eye exercises

1. Screw the eyes up as tight as possible, then open them wide, simultaneously pushing out the tongue.

2. Keeping the head still, look as far as you can to the right. Count to five. Bring the vision back to the centre and then look as far as you can to the left. Count to five. Repeat five times.

Keeping the head still, look down as far as you can. Count to five. Bring the vision back to the centre, then look up as far as you can. Count to five. Repeat five times.

3. Repeat the first exercise, combining the movement with a neck stretch to the right, looking as far as you can around the back, repeat to the left, co-ordinating the movements with the breath.

Repeat the second exercise, combining the eye movements with neck stretches forward and backward; try to look at your chin as you bend the head forward, and over the head as you bend the head back.

4. Focus on the tip of a pen bringing it towards you until it it a few inches away from the tip of your nose. Count to three. Shift your focus to an object in the distance, as far away as possible; count to three. Repeat twenty times.

● Sun-bathing and moon-gazing:

A little book I bought in India suggests that sun-bathing and moon-gazing benefit the eyes. Sitting or standing in a relaxed position, face the sun with the eyes closed. Gently move the head from side to side.

When the moon is full, lie in a comfortable position and blink the eyes while gazing at the moon. Keep the eyes relaxed. Practise for ten minutes.

• Watching TV

The same little book gives instructions on how best to watch TV and states categorically that children under the age of 12 should not be allowed to watch TV for more than a short time each day. With TV, videos and computers becoming more and more a part of our everyday lives and education system, we need to take some compensatory measures to help our children's eyes. While constant exposure to the screen obviously has adverse effects on everyone's eyesight, it is more pronounced with children, as their eyes have not completely grown and developed.

INSOMNIA

There are three categories of insomnia, which involve the basic balance of yin and yang, fire and water in the body. They are: over-stimulation of the mind, long-term insomnia and disrupted sleep patterns.

CALMING THE MIND

Symptoms:
• Too much thinking, cannot turn off
• Difficulty going off to sleep

Over-stimulation of the mind is the most common kind of insomnia; in Chinese medicine it is considered to be an imbalance of the heart. This may be a short-term problem, and over-stimulation of the mind in the evening – attending meetings, presenting talks or studying late into the night – frequently results in the inability to turn off and sleep. This is quite natural and may be helped by performing certain relaxing techniques before going to bed.

If the inability to sleep is prolonged, it may be helpful to examine the thoughts that are going around in your head. Are they real worries, or is your mind just flitting from one thing to another? Is your inability to sleep rooted from real-life problems that need to be addressed, or is your mind just unable to settle?

Once the body forgets its natural rhythms it needs help to get them re-established. And again it is the regularity here that is important.

Treatment:

As with all heart problems, the most effective method of treatment is with meditation and breathing exercises. This type of insomnia is differentiated from the next by being specifically related to problems in initially getting off to sleep. If you tend to wake in the middle of the night, the cause is more likely to be with the kidneys, and the suggestions made there will be more helpful. Insomnia is usually a problem of fire–water imbalance or heart and kidney imbalance in the body; depending on the type of insomnia, it is better to begin treatment with the heart or the kidneys.

These exercises can be carried out in a sitting position before going to bed, or while lying down. Take care that the spine is straight and the body relaxed. Insomnia, as we saw with headaches, is due to an excess of yang energy in the head. The body is tired but the mind cannot turn off. It is important to remove the concentration from the head and to bring the awareness into the lower abdomen.

• Calming the heart by regulating the breathing

Sitting comfortably with the back straight, or lying down with the head raised on a small pillow, focus the mind on the breath. Make sure that the armpits are slightly open and that the arms are not too close to the sides of the body; feel that the chest has plenty of space to expand sideways, and that air can circulate freely in the armpits. Placing the hands with the palms upwards on the knees or in the lap naturally brings the arms into the correct position. Relax the shoulders.

Feel the air as it moves gently through the nostrils, the gentle expansion and contraction of the ribcage. Concentrating the mind completely on the breath, begin counting slowly to four with each inhalation, and to four with each exhalation. Repeat for five minutes.

● Relaxing the muscles

Lying on your back in bed, contract the muscles of the body and then release. Repeat three times. Make sure that you are warm enough, as cold stops the muscles relaxing.

Slowly work through the body, first contracting and releasing the toes, the feet, the calves, the thighs, the hands, the arms, the shoulders. Allow the feet to fall away from the centre, the hands to lie palm up. Relax the eyes, the ears, the tongue. Relax the brain. Feel the head to be heavy on the pillow. Breathe deeply and evenly.

● Concentrating on the lower abdomen

Close your eyes and move the attention to the lower abdomen as if you are withdrawing your sight from the outside world and looking within. Be gentle, do not force it as this immediately activates the brain and introduces tension. Imagine that you are breathing into the lower abdomen, feel the abdomen gently rise and fall with the breath. If you feel more comfortable, bring your hands to rest over the abdomen. Focusing on the lower abdomen, count the breaths from one to ten.

● Developing a routine

When possible, try to develop a routine for winding down. In the same way that we teach children a sleeping routine, we often have to re-educate our own bodies when they lose their natural rhythms. As much as possible avoid mental stimulation at night; even watching television tends to over-stimulate the brain and the eyes, and if you are prone to insomnia try to avoid watching TV for a couple of hours before you go to bed. Listen to music. Try taking a walk in the evening as gentle movement helps the body relax, release tension and restore natural rhythms. Have a hot bath in candlelight with relaxing bath oils. Lavender is often a favourite.

If none of the above seems to help, it may be that the cause of the problem is with the kidney energy. We have seen that the heart and the kidney energy must be in balance, as it is easy for the fire of the heart to become out of control if not tempered by the water of the kidneys.

STRENGTHENING THE KIDNEYS

Symptoms:
• Long term insomnia
• Waking up in the middle of the night
• Night sweats

In the case of long-term insomnia it is always wise to strengthen the kidneys, and this is essential if you tend to wake up in the middle of the night and find it difficult to go back to sleep or if you suffer from night sweats. Waking up in the middle of the night may be accompanied by the need to pass urine.

The kidneys are said to root the energy in the depths of the body, particularly at night. If the kidneys are weak, they are unable to hold the energy down and it literally floats up. The eyes open and you are awake. A common time for this waking is around four or five a.m. when, according to the traditional measurement of energy in the acupuncture meridians, the kidney energy is at its lowest. In more severe cases you may find that you suddenly wake up as soon as a deep level of sleep is reached.

Treatment:
The cause of kidney depletion is very often long-term exhaustion and overwork. Exhaustion may be mental or emotional as well as physical, and the Chinese consider excessive sex to be one of the main causes of kidney depletion for men. An indication that sexual patterns are excessive is feeling exhausted after intercourse. For women kidney depletion is traditionally associated with problems in pregnancy and childbirth, or too many pregnancies in quick succession. All these problems require serious attention and possibly adjustment of lifestyle patterns. In severe kidney depletion the best treatment is rest.

• Massage the soles of the feet and Kidney 1
Massage the sole of the foot with the thumbs, as described on p. 123, No. 3. Massage each foot for at least three minutes (Fig. 14).

● Massage Kidney 3, Stomach 36
Apply gentle circular movements with the thumbs over the points Kidney 3, just behind the inner ankle bone, and Stomach 36, below the knee. In this case massage is preferable to moxa, as moxa can cause too much heat and create a yang response (Figs 117 and 118).

● Lower abdominal breathing
In this case lower abdominal breathing is performing not just to move the concentration from the head but to strengthen the kidneys. It can be performed, as suggested above, before going to bed, but to strengthen the kidneys it is best also practised during the day when the energy levels are higher.

Sitting with the spine straight, close your eyes and move the attention to the lower abdomen. Concentrate the mind on the lower abdomen and breathe deeply and regularly. Feel the abdomen gently expanding and contracting with the inhalation and the exhalation. When the breath is stable and you are easily able to keep the concentration in the abdominal area, breathe in more deeply, holding the breath for a few seconds as you contract the muscles of the perineum. Relax the muscles as you exhale. Repeat to a count of 20 breaths. Do not force and do not hold the breath for more than a few seconds. This action helps to strengthen the lower abdominal energy.

● Herbal remedy Liu wei di huang wan
When there is long-term depletion of the yin of the body resulting in lack of blood, lack of nutrition, lack of fluids, lack of essence, herbal remedies are very effective and can be safely used over extended periods. The Chinese herbal remedy Liu wei di huang wan, or six-flavour tea, is a classical formula to treat kidney weakness and can be used very effectively in this kind of insomnia.

BALANCING YIN AND YANG QIAO MAI

Symptoms:
● Sleep patterns disrupted

- Jet lag
- Working unusual hours

When discussing the extraordinary meridians, we saw how the yin and yang qiao mai are involved in the balance of energy between day and night, sleeping and waking. Working with this energy cycle can be particularly helpful if the sleep patterns have been disrupted by extended travelling or working shifts, and if natural cycles have been disrupted as they often are in types of Chronic Fatigue Syndrome.

Treament:
The aim here is to restore rhythm and regularity to the system and to balance yin and yang. Many of the basic qi gong exercises will be effective, but we will look at a few specific variations. Read the section on the yin and yang qiao mai (pp. 87–90) to refresh your memory.

- Circulation of light – breathing through the heels
The Daoist meditation 'the circulation of light' is generally described as following the pathways of the governor vessel (du mai) and conception vessel (ren mai), but it can also be performed by imagining the breath is coming from the heels. This activates the yin and yang qiao mai which both have their beginnings in the heels. The yin qiao passes up the inner part of the leg and the front of the body, the yang qiao over the outer part of the leg and the back. They both meet at the eyes.

This circulation can be visualised while practising the basic qi gong exercise, drawing the energy up through the yin qiao to the lower abdomen and straight up to the head, and back through the yang qiao over the back of the head, and down through the backs of the legs.

Otherwise it may be visualised while sitting or standing still. In cases of insomnia it is important to imagine that the yin energy is being drawn up through the feet to the head, the yang energy down from the head to the feet. This helps to restore the natural rhythm of sleeping and waking.

• Walking

The relationship of yin qiao mai and yang qiao mai to the heels and the ankles means that this circulation is stimulated when walking. This is referred to in some of the ancient medical texts. The rhythm and pace of the walking is important in restoring a good balance between these two extraordinary meridians and therefore between yin and yang.

• Attempt to restore regularity and rhythm

You can help to restore the rhythm of waking and sleeping by restoring the other rhythms of your life. Eating regular meals can begin to set the body back into a natural cycle. And as always, pay attention to the regularity of the breath.

BREATHING PROBLEMS

STRENGTHENING THE LUNGS

Symptoms:
• Shortness of breath
• Constriction in the chest
• Difficult to exhale
• Skin problems

All breathing problems will respond to breathing exercise, but if your lungs are weak and your lung capacity restricted, work slowly and carefully, do not attempt to hold the breath. Follow the exercises described on pp. 189–193.

Treatment:
• Breathing and qi gong exercises
• Lung qi gong

WORKING WITH THE KIDNEYS

Symptoms:
• Breathlessness on exertion

- Breathing fast and weak
- Difficulty in inhaling
- Cold weak back

We have seen that some cases of insomnia may be caused by weakness of the kidney energy, and the same is true with breathing difficulties. In a similar way, the kidneys cannot root the energy in the lower part of the body, which leads to congestion in the chest. This is particularly the case in inherited weaknesses and breathing problems in young children. Of course the lungs are also involved, but there is often little long-term improvement unless the kidneys are also strengthened.

You would expect to see some other signs of kidney weakness, for example lack of energy or breathing difficulties on exertion. There may be coldness or aching in the lower back and, as with all kidney-based problems, it is vital to keep this area warm. Once the kidney energy is strengthened the lungs will immediately begin to improve.

Treatments:
- Breathing to the lower abdomen
Sitting or lying down with the spine straight, follow the exercise described on p. 216.

- Warming the kidneys
Rub the hands together and place them over the kidneys. Repeat three times. Massage gently, stimulating the circulation in the lower back. Make sure that you are warm, wearing extra layers if necessary to protect the vital kidney points (Fig. 120).

- Moxa to Ren 6
Heat the acupuncture point sea of qi (Ren 6) with a moxa stick or stick-on moxa cones. The stick is very effective in this area as it is not necessary to be precise (Fig. 116).

- Moxa to Kidney 3
Heat the acupuncture point Kidney 3, beside the inner ankle bone, preferably with stick-on moxa cones. This point stimulates the energy of the kidneys. Use three cones (Fig. 121).

• Herbal remedy Ping chuan wan
This is a traditional herbal formula for treating chronic breathing problems with associated kidney weakness. It strengthens the qi, and helps to stop coughs as well as strengthening the kidneys. It can be safely used for prolonged periods.

CHILDHOOD ASTHMA

Symptoms:
• Tightness in the chest
• Wheezing
• Often accompanied or preceded by eczema
• May occur after immunisation

I hesitated to introduce childhood asthma here, but it is an area where we can begin to extend the simple concepts of self-help to our families. Childhood asthma is increasing at an alarming rate. Alternative medical practitioners have long suspected that the increase in childhood immunisation may have played a major part and, along with the issue of pollutants and allergens, this is now being taken seriously by the orthodox medical profession. The over-prescription of anti-asthma drugs, especially inhalers, has been shown to decrease long-term recovery, so alternative methods of alleviating breathlessness are essential.

Treatment:
Although it may be useful to see a qualified Chinese medical doctor for long-term treatment of problems such as asthma and eczema, there are many things that can be done in the home.

• Diet
Many childhood outbreaks of asthma and eczema are a direct result of allergy to cow's milk. This kind of allergy often occurs soon after weaning, as the child is introduced to a variety of foods. It is always worth trying a complete break from dairy produce to see if this helps the condition. This

kind of pathology is rarely mentioned in traditional Chinese books, and many Chinese and Japanese doctors will not be aware of this as a possible irritant, as traditionally Chinese and Japanese diets contain very little dairy produce.

● Massage and warm upper back
Keep the muscles in the upper back loose by massage. Gentle rubbing will be sufficient in small babies. All asthma will be helped by regular massage of the upper back. In many cases the asthma involves the lung energy only, and is not accompanied by lack of energy or weight loss. But if this is the case, steps should also be taken to strengthen the kidneys.

● Massage and warm the kidney area
In cases of early childhood asthma there is very often a weakness in the kidneys, possibly an inherited weakness, or one caused during pregnancy. As we saw when we looked at the lower heater, the kidneys are the basis for the deep defensive energies of the body. Immunisations, especially when carried out on the very young, can interfere with the development of the immune system and also with the energy of the kidneys. Although the kidney energy is difficult to build when damaged so young, there is much that can be done to stop further depletion and to help the body make the most of what is available. As we have seen many times, the kidneys need warmth. And as the kidney meridian flows through the soles of the feet it is particularly important for the feet to be kept warm. Being warm and well nourished are the two prerequisites to develop kidney energy and a healthy immune system. Rub the kidney area with the palm, warming the hands first by rubbing them vigorously together.

DIGESTIVE PROBLEMS

STRENGTHENING THE SPLEEN

Symptoms:
● Lack of energy

- Limbs feel cold
- Tendency to put on weight, or to lose weight
- Diarrhoea with undigested food in stool
- Feeling of heaviness in the limbs

Spleen weakness is often accompanied by tiredness and a heaviness in the limbs. There is a lack of the basic transformation and transportation of the spleen energy and, as we have seen, this may manifest as weight gain or weight loss.

Treatments:
Most of these treatments have been covered under the section on the earth element and the spleen (pp. 193–200) and we will just give a brief reminder here.

- Moxa to Stomach 36, Spleen 6
The acupuncture points Stomach 36 and Spleen 6 are the most powerful points to stimulate the transforming power of the earth element. Use stick-on moxa cones on both points on both legs. Rotate, burning one cone on one point and moving on to the next. Repeat three times on each point (Figs 103–4).

- Eat warm foods
When the spleen is deficient it needs warm foods. Rather than salads or raw vegetables, make soups and stir-fries. This helps the body to assimilate the energy from food, which often means that you need to eat less. Cooked food is also less likely to be passed through the body without being broken down, as is often the case with weight loss from spleen deficiency.

- Eat regularly
Regularity is probably the most important factor in healthy eating. Skipping meals, or snacking between meals, confuses the system and can create chaos if it becomes the normal pattern of behaviour. As we have seen, all these autonomic or unconscious activities of the body like nothing more than rhythm and regularity. The secretions of digestive juices and the hormones that aid assimilation function well when they

are given these conditions. The spleen is described as the revolving centre of the body, always there, always working and we can greatly aid its function by giving it the regularity it needs to perform well.

● Abdominal massage

Massaging the abdomen, always in a clockwise direction, is another way to help the digestive processes of the spleen. This is particularly the case if you feel tightness above the navel which is often associated with stress. Try to relax and breathe deeply for a few minutes before eating, and with the right hand over the left make circular stroking movements around the navel. If there is tightness above the navel try making smaller circular movements with the heel of the hand in this area (Fig. 105). You may hear gurgling and rumbling which is often a sign of the release of tension.

● Avoid damp

The spleen dislikes dampness, and clinically many cases of severe spleen depletion can be traced back to living in damp conditions. If the body is strong, you should be able to cope with occasional exposure to damp without any ill effects, but if you suspect this to be an area of weakness for you, it is worth taking particular care. Make sure that you dry properly after taking a bath; avoid sitting on damp ground. If you are living in a house that tends to be damp, air it as much as you can, and make sure that your bed is in the driest possible position.

Living in damp conditions can undermine the transformational power of the spleen, affecting the transformation and reabsorption of fluids. The result is often the over-production of phlegm and mucus, which eventually affects the lungs. Many severe spleen and lung problems of this kind can be completely cured by moving to a less damp environment, and sometimes this may be the only effective solution. In the UK our houses often tend to be old and made of porous materials that hold the damp; as the climate is also damp, these kinds of problems tend to be very common in the UK and we need to be particularly careful to take care of our spleen energy.

BALANCING THE LIVER AND SPLEEN

Symptoms:
- Nausea
- Vomiting
- Bitter taste in the mouth
- Belching

Whereas digestive problems due to spleen deficiency are often accompanied by lethargy or loss of energy, the imbalance of the liver and the spleen is more a problem of excess and, as we so often find with the liver, a problem of an excessive liver energy invading the spleen. The symptoms may be violent but are often short-lived, though this kind of imbalance is also at the root of much nausea and vomiting in pregnancy.

Nausea may also be present in spleen deficiency patterns, but here it is usually accompanied by a feeling of fullness and abdominal distention, a bitter taste in the mouth and relief from belching.

Treatment:
- Massage Liver 3
The acupuncture point Liver 3 (Fig. 114), in the depression on the top of the foot between the big toe and the second toe, calms excessive liver energy. You may also stimulate the energy of the stomach and spleen by using moxa on Stomach 36, but it is best if this is done after calming the liver.

- Herbal remedy Xiao yao wan
The Chinese herbal remedy Xiao yao wan (also known as Relaxed Wanderer) is a classical formula which has been used for centuries to calm aggressive liver energy.

- Exercise
When experiencing this kind of discomfort, moving often brings improvement, and any of the stretches suggested to free the liver energy will be useful – especially as a preventive measure. If you are experiencing nausea, gentle side stretches or walking while swinging the arms will help to free stuck liver qi.

INVIGORATING THE INTESTINES

Symptoms:
- Abdominal gas
- Constipation
- Alternating constipation and diarrhoea

Many of the symptoms that we would generally associate with the intestines are treated by the spleen in Chinese medicine. Intestinal problems tend to be less chronic and the suggestions below are particularly effective for constipation.

Treatment:
- Abdominal massage

Massage the abdomen in a clockwise direction, following the course of the large intestine (Fig. 122). This stimulates the necessary muscular action to expel the stool. Fifty rotations first thing in the morning and last thing at night are recommended to help move the bowels. The points Stomach 25, the main treatment point of the large intestine, and Ren 4 (gate to the origin), the main treatment point for the small intestine, should be included in this massage (Fig. 123).

- Massaging point Large intestine 4

This acupuncture point on the hand is frequently used for all kinds of pain relief. It is a major point for 'letting go', and this applies especially to the stress and tension in the bowels as well as to any other area. It is an important relaxing and releasing point. Activate it by pressing with the thumb, and massaging in small circles. Do not use moxa (Fig. 124).

MENSTRUAL DISORDERS

The menstrual cycle is a good indicator of your general energetic tendencies, and information about the cycle is used by all Chinese doctors as an aid in diagnosis. This natural cycle is one way in which women are able to tune in to their

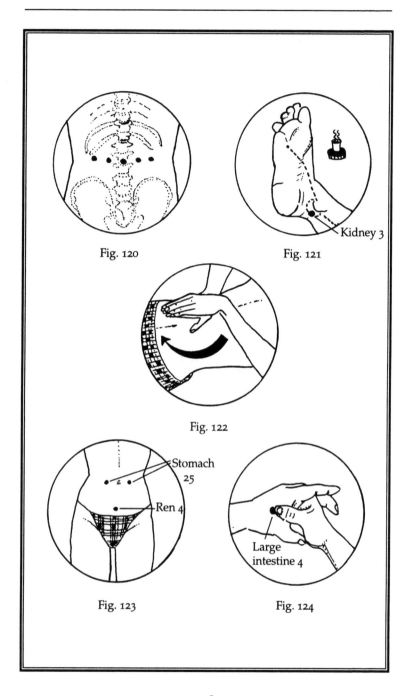

Fig. 120

Fig. 121

Kidney 3

Fig. 122

Stomach 25

Ren 4

Fig. 123

Large intestine 4

Fig. 124

bodies more easily than men – they already have a guide, a reminder of the cyclical natural of energy.

Many women come to see an acupuncturist for complaints unrelated to menstruation, but find that as a result of the treatment their cycles become regular, and their periods become less painful. Practising the general qi gong cycles for balancing heaven and earth or the basic meridian stretches will help to balance the meridians and the internal organs and many period problems will be regulated. Practising with regularity helps to create regularity in the body.

In my clinical practice I often ask patients with menstrual problems to come at a specific time of the month, and aim to maintain fortnightly treatments – often treating at the end of the cycle to restore blood, and premenstrually to aid the free-flow of blood. A similar system can be followed with your own self-treatments, depending on your individual symptoms.

Menstruation involves the three yin meridians in the legs, the kidneys, spleen and liver (these three meridians all meet in the centre of the lower abdomen just above the pubic bone at points Ren 3 and 4), and also the extraordinary meridians ren mai, chong mai and dai mai, though the functions of these extraordinary meridians are often treated by activating the kidney, spleen and liver meridians respectively.

Many menstrual problems are caused by tension in the lower abdomen and a lack of nourishment by the three yin meridians involved. One simple exercise is beneficial for all menstrual problems and can be practised during the period to alleviate pain as well as at other times to relax the pelvic and abdominal muscles generally and stimulate the spleen, liver and kidney meridians. You will need some pillows to support your back.

Exercise:
Sitting with the feet pulled up towards the groin, allow the knees to fall out to the side. Support them with cushions so that you can feel a slight stretch but the legs are able to relax. You can begin with the cushions under the thighs and as your groin muscles begin to relax, move them out towards the knees. Lie back with pillows under your back and head. Feel

that your spine is straight and slightly stretched, the back of the neck long, your chin tucked in. Be aware of the contact between your sacrum and the floor. Relax the sacrum, feel it releasing and widening. Bring the hands to the lower abdomen and rest them just above the pubic bone (covering points Ren 3 and 4). Breathe deeply, releasing tension around the groin and lower abdomen as you breathe out (Fig. 125). Rest in this position for at least ten minutes.

DEFICIENCY OF BLOOD

Symptoms:
- Light flow
- Light colour
- Late start, short duration
- Stops and starts
- Dragging pain during period
- Deficiency headaches after period

Blood is yin, and a lack of blood is a yin deficiency. It can therefore best be treated successfully on the main yin meridian, the conception vessel or ren mai. A deficiency of yin suggests a need for nourishment on all levels, including diet and rest.

Treatments:
- Eat regularly and well
Nourishing ourselves during a period is very important, especially if the period tends to be scanty and is often late. Warm foods such as soups and stews provide a feeling of well-being and inner warmth – and it is important during menstruation to feel as if you are pampering yourself, looking after yourself. You can create special dishes which you reserve for this time, using roots such as carrots, parsnips and sweet potatoes to nourish the yin in warming casseroles with aduki beans to strengthen the kidneys. If you eat meat, you may add some red meat to your diet before your period; lamb is particularly warming. Give yourself and your diet a bit more attention than usual.

• Rest after eating

It is always beneficial to rest after eating, but if you are trying to build up your blood and help a painful period, this is vital.

• Rest as much as possible during a period

It is not fashionable to treat ourselves differently during menstruation. Advertisements encourage us to keep up our active lives and carry on as normal. Peer pressure and embarrassment during teenage years may set a pattern for life. Painful, scanty periods often show inner tensions around bleeding, and if we pretend to ourselves that nothing is happening, problems become worse. Something is happening – and if we make allowances, our bodies will respond by relaxing and releasing in a natural way. Allow your body to rest and relax. If you really want to play a game of tennis, then that's fine, but make sure that the desire is coming from your body, not from your mind.

• Keep the abdomen warm

Coldness contracts, and contraction causes more pain. This kind of yin depletion responds well to warmth – and the pain may be alleviated with a hot-water bottle on the lower back or on the lower abdomen. But most important – wear enough clothes, keep the kidney area warm, and keep the feet warm.

• Moxa to Ren 3 and 4

Use stick-on moxa cones or a moxa stick to stimulate the points Ren 3 (central axis) and Ren 4 (gate to the origin). These are the main points in the lower abdomen to tonify the blood and the yin (Fig. 126).

If you do not have moxa, create warmth in the abdomen with your hands. First rub them vigorously together and then place your hands palms down over the lower part of the abdomen. Concentrate your mind on the points and imagine that the nourishment of the earth is flowing up through your legs and permeating the lower abdomen, releasing tension and strengthening the flow.

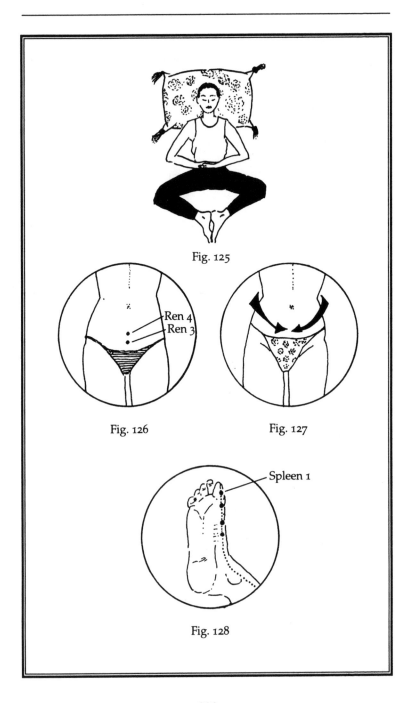

Fig. 125

Ren 4
Ren 3

Fig. 126

Fig. 127

Spleen 1

Fig. 128

● Herbal remedy Dang gui, or Eight Treasure Tea
The classical herbal formulas are particularly safe and effective in helping yin deficiency problems. Dang gui (Chinese angelica) is a single herb used to build up the blood and is given to women in China after childbirth or any loss of blood. It may be taken effectively after the period to build up after the loss of blood. Dang gui is also used in Eight Treasure Tea, or Women's Precious formula, where it is combined with other herbs to strengthen the qi. This formula is particularly useful taken in the two weeks before the period, both to build the blood and to promote the flow.

PREMENSTRUAL TENSION

Symptoms:
● Irritability
● Headaches
● Swelling of the breasts
● Abdominal pain

Premenstrual tension is one of the most common signs of liver stagnation in women, a time when all those suppressed emotions come up into the light of day to be examined. There are many ways we can begin to address the build-up of tension, but perhaps we should also give ourselves the chance to listen to some of our grievances. We may be over-emotional, but maybe this is the only time we allow these inner feelings any expression. What are they telling us? Begin to see your feelings as symbols of inner conflict. If we feel we want to kill our husbands, maybe what we really want is to kill that over-critical male part of ourselves that does not allow us to be at one with our bodies.

Treatment:
● Aiding freeflow of the liver
The most effective way to aid the freeflow of the liver is to allow the emotions free expression: learning to watch the flow of the emotions without totally engaging, becom-

ing an observer, not repressing and not suppressing but allowing.

● Walking
Walking during the days before the period can help the regulation of the flow and keep the liver energy circulating well. Use the breath, and try to get a good rhythm into your walk.

● Gentle side stretches
Stand with the arms by the sides, knees straight and feet parallel hip-width apart. With the out-breath slide the right hand down the right leg allowing that movement to pull the body over to the right. Feel the stretch at the side of the ribcage. This is the area which often becomes stagnant when the liver qi is not flowing well. Repeat to the left. If you have pains in the breasts, stretch the arm gently over the head as you repeat the stretch to the right and left. Always work gently with the breath, stretching as you breathe out, returning to the centre as you breathe in (Figs. 91, 92).

● Invigorating dai mai
Dai mai controls the flow of energy between the top and the bottom of the body. It flows from the area of the kidneys at the back of the waist around under the ribcage and descends into the lower abdomen. Lack of freeflow in the abdominal area may be a symptom of a constriction of dai mai.

Rub the hands together until they are warm and place them over the kidneys. Repeat three times. Massage using the heels of the hands with a stroking movement along the pathway of dai mai – begin with the hands over the kidneys, and end with the hands together over the lower abdomen. Repeat ten times (Fig. 127).

● Herbal remedy Xiao yao wan
The herbal formula Xiao yao wan, or the Relaxed Wanderer, frees liver stagnation by building the blood and yin of the liver. As with many of these classical formulas it consists of a carefully balanced selection of herbs which make it safe even

in long-term use. Many women find that in taking Xiao yao wan for two weeks before menstruation they alleviate many premenstrual problems and regulate the menstrual cycle. If you feel exhausted after the period and also suffer from premenstrual tension, try taking Xiao yao wan for two weeks before the period and Women's Precious for a week or so after the period.

HEAVY PERIODS

Symptoms:
● Heavy bleeding
● Blood may be dark with clots

Heavy periods are often an indication of spleen weakness related to the function of the spleen to hold the blood, possibly involving over-activity of the liver as well, especially if there is premenstrual tension and strong period pains. If there is heavy bleeding with exhaustion, but not so much pain, then concentrate on strengthening the spleen.

Treatment:
● Moxa cones to Spleen 6 and Stomach 36
If the spleen is not able to hold the blood, the earth needs to be strengthened. During the two weeks leading up to the period use moxa treatment on the points Spleen 6 and Stomach 36 (Figs 103–4). Use three cones on each point in rotation, 12 cones in all. Treat every three days until the period begins. Moxa should not be used during the period as heat can cause a heavier flow.

● Strengthen the spleen with massage
Massage the spleen meridian from Spleen 1 to Spleen 4 (Fig. 128). In the bath you can use a loofah or Japanese washing cloth to stimulate this area, where a build-up of dead skin can often make the circulation sluggish. Spleen 1, at the outside edge of the base of the big toenail, is an acupuncture point

often used in haemorrhage, and can be stimulated with your fingernail as an emergency treatment.

● Avoid hot foods
Excess heat can aggravate the symptoms of heavy bleeding. To keep away from hot foods does not mean food with a hot temperature, but with a hot energy, for example spices, alcohol, red meat and greasy food.

MENOPAUSE

Symptoms:
● Hot flushes
● Yin deficiency in the upper body
● Yang deficiency in the lower body

The symptoms associated with menopause are many and varied, and here we will look at the basic pattern of imbalance according to the theory of yin and yang. As we saw on p. 29, at seven times six years the yin no longer reaches the head and the eyes, the eyesight begins to decline, and the face to wrinkle, the hair becomes dry; at seven times seven years the text says that the conception vessel (ren mai) dries up, the great penetrating vessel (chong mai) declines, and a woman can no longer have children.

This is a natural process and Chinese medicine has no answers for keeping menopause at bay – only to make it a natural life-enhancing transition. As the body ages, the yin can no longer easily reach the head, the yang no longer bring its enlivening energies to the lower abdomen. Within the Chinese medical framework we can aid this in many ways.

● Balancing yin and yang
Qi gong for balancing yin and yang is very effective. Use your full concentration to feel the nourishment of the earth being drawn up through your body, the vitalising yang being pulled down from above. Establish a good rhythm in your movement, encouraging new energetic cycles. Take time to contact

the lower abdomen, the gate to the origin, bringing the earth and heaven together, weaving the yin and yang to form a new web of life. Feel at one with the earth and at one with heaven.

In meditation, imagine that you are drawing up yin nourishment from the earth and bringing it to the head, and drawing yang energy down from heaven and bringing it into the lower abdomen. Work with the breath.

● Balancing fire and water

Many problems of heat and excess are due to a lack of fluid, a lack of the cooling and stabilising effect of the yin of the kidneys. The hot flushes and palpitations associated with menopause are typical of this kind of 'false heat' and come from the natural decline of the yin of the kidneys at this time. Herbs to build the yin provide a more natural solution to the false perpetuation of periods which ultimately leads to more yin deficiency through prolonged loss of blood.

Many Chinese herbal formulas for menopause are now available, and you should consult a trained herbalist if your symptoms are severe, as herbs can be combined in many ways to suit your individual pattern of disharmony. As a general kidney yin tonic Liu wei di huang wan is very effective, and can be used in the long term, particularly as a preventive treatment if taken at the first signs of alteration to your cycle.

● Healthy bones and joints

The sequence of exercises to stimulate the flow of qi in the meridians works on all the joints and ensures a good blood supply to the bones and muscles. These exercises were performed by elderly women in Japan over a period of six months or so with marked improvement to their mobility. They are also recommended to prevent bone degeneration. If there is a good blood supply to all parts of the body, the necessary nutrients will be distributed.

JOINT PROBLEMS

The exercises to invigorate the meridian system are designed to keep the joints supple and to prevent joint problems. The acupuncture meridians have a special relationship with the joints, often binding around them and sending internal pathways through them; many of the vital and most commonly used acupuncture points are found here. Chinese medicine theory teaches us that energy tends to stagnate in the joints, and advises that we take care to keep the joints moving. If you have pain, go carefully. Be gentle with the body at all times. If the degree of pain and stiffness means that movement is difficult, do a little – but imagine the complete movement, visualising it in your mind. If the fingers are stiff, stretch them as much as you can, but with your imagination visualise the fingers stretching, the energy projecting as far as the horizon. Gently pull the fingers and massage the fingertips. Once the energy begins to move, the joints will slowly free up. It may take time – but keep at it, working gently and persistently until the movement becomes easier.

Chinese medicine is often successful with arthritis and general aches and pains in the joints because it classifies them according to the energies of the five elements, as hot or cold, contracted or swollen, or moving and changing.

Cold joints can be warmed with a moxa stick and respond well to massage and movement. But if the joints are hot and swollen, they must be treated with care, and may be aggravated by heat and motion. Do not work on an inflamed joint but try to help the flow of energy through the area. If the wrist is hot and swollen, massage the fingers and squeeze them at the base of the nails. All the meridians have their 'well' points at the tips of the fingers and toes and the whole meridian can be stimulated by massaging these points. By stimulating the energy to move through the area of stagnation, the heat and swelling can begin to disperse. In cases of severe heat and pain, acupuncture treatment is effective.

Heat suggests an involvement of the fire element, the heart and the circulation system. Moving pains imply liver wind. Swelling suggests dampness and a weakness of the spleen.

Tightness with grinding may suggest a lack of fluid and the over-activity of the metal element; coldness may imply a weakness of the kidney energy. As well as working on the individual joint with massage and exercise, try to strengthen the associated element and organ by looking over the appropriate sections above.

CONCLUSION

Looking back, I am aware of many oversimplifications and oversights, and have to remind myself constantly that I am not writing a textbook. For those who would like more detailed and precise information, many such books exist. What I hope to have achieved is an introduction to a medical system that is rich in metaphor and symbolism, full of simple wisdom and insight which may help to lead us back to our body-knowing.

Many of the ideas appear childish and simplistic, and yet they work. We are talking body language here, and although our intellect may cry out that this is not enough – our bodies respond by expanding and letting go.

Our bodies know what they need, but we have forgotten how to listen to them. Once we begin to listen to our bodies and trust our feelings, we can also begin to work with health professionals in co-operation and partnership, no longer 'the doctor as expert' but the doctor as partner in a process of understanding and cure. As patients we have given away our power and it is up to us to claim it back. As practitioners we have assumed an overwhelming responsibility that is not ours to take.

If we can slow down and tune in with our body rhythms, we can realign with the healing power of nature; no longer fearing or needing to control nature – but observing and learning from nature. By observing heaven and earth we can begin to understand yin and yang; by observing yin and yang as it manifests in the four seasons, we can begin to understand the movements of the five elements. By tuning in to the cycles of the seasons and the cycles of our lives we can begin to reclaim the wisdom of the body.

FURTHER READING

For an introduction to Chinese medicine:
A Guide to Acupuncture by Peter Firebrace and Sandra Hill,
  Constable, London (1993)

For more detailed information on the concepts presented in
Parts 1 and 2: 'Chinese Medicine from the Classics' a series
published by Monkey Press, Cambridge, on the work of
Claude Larre and Elisabeth Rochat de la Vallée: *The Spleen
and Stomach* (1990), *The Heart* (1991), *The Heart Master and
Triple Heater* (1992), *The Kidneys* (1992), *The Lung* (1992), *The
Secret Treatise of the Spiritual Orchid* (1992), *The Liver* (1994),
The Way of Heaven (1994), *The Seven Emotions* (1996), *The Eight
Extraordinary Meridians* (1997).

For more information on the work of Hiroshi Motoyama:
Theories of the Chakras, Quest Books, Wheaton, IL (1981)
Toward a Superconsciousness, Asian Humanities Press, Berke-
  ley, CA (1990)
Karma and Reincarnation, Piatkus, London (1992)
A Study of Yoga from Eastern and Western Medical Viewpoints,
  Human Science Press, Tokyo (1993)

Practical workbooks:
Self Massage by Jaqueline Young, Thorsons, London (1992)
Acupressure for Health by Jaqueline Young, Thorsons, London
  (1994)

INDEX

abdomen, 62, 64, 84, 183, 198, 225, 227
231, 233; *see also* lower abdomen;
upper abdomen
acupuncture, 2–3, 4, 6, 28, 59, 60;
meridians, 70, 100, 119, 238; points, 62,
66, 72–93, 151, 155, 176, 196; scientific
explanations of, 61
addictions, 44, 54, 195
aggressive liver energy, 208–10, 226
agitation, 19, 34, 36, 37, 94, 159
Agpaoa, Tony, 165
alchemy, 21, 28, 52, 59, 72, 94, 97
alcohol, 38, 54
alternate nostril breathing, 155–6
ancestral qi, 81, 102
anger, 19, 34, 35, 37, 43, 45–6, 48, 50, 110,
178, 179, 181, 182, 196, 208
ankles, 88, 119, 121, 132, 220
armpit, 113, 142, 165, 167, 168, 190, 215
arms, 62, 64, 135, 144, 167
artemisa vulgaris *see* moxa/moxibustion
arthritis, 119, 238
artistic expression, 179–80
asthma, 20, 47, 103, 187, 222–3
astral projection, 50, 51, 52
attention, focusing the, 116–18
autumn, 14, 16, 17, 18, 20, 40, 41, 46, 118,
163, 187

back, 69, 76, 143, 221, 223
bai hui *see* one hundred meetings
balance, 13, 17, 21, 27, 68, 87–93, 112,
203–8, 214, 236–7; of left and right
sides, 140–8, 150–1
basic prone position, 143, 148
bearing, 77–8
belching, 226
benevolence, 180
birth, 45–6
bladder, 20, 30, 64, 65, 90, 94, 100, 120,
123, 129, 135, 140, 144, 155, 173, 175,
176, 204, 205, 213
blockage, 19, 34, 35, 47, 48, 84, 87
blood, 6, 19, 21, 22, 23, 31–2, 34, 35–6, 38,
51–2, 78, 81, 84, 91, 101–2, 159, 229,
230, 235
body, 26, 27, 39, 54, 81, 91, 111, 240–1;
and five elements, 19–21; and heaven
and earth, 13–14; landscape of, 62; left
and right sides, 140–8, 150–1; and

subtle energies, 59–61; sweeping
exercise, 140
body-knowing, 2, 5, 14, 98
body swings, 182–3
bones, 27, 29, 54, 74, 237
bowels, 189, 227
brain, 27, 54, 72, 74, 76, 150, 205, 207
breast problems, 185
breath, 39, 52, 76, 81, 101, 108, 142, 144,
151, 152, 155–6, 187, 193; counting the,
155, 156, 167, 169–70, 190, 207;
regulating the, 167–8, 189, 215, 220; *see
also* breathing
breathing, 5, 25, 39, 47, 53, 81, 104, 113,
120; alternate nostrils, 155–6; in lower
abdomen, 218, 221; problems, 220–3;
shallow, 188; through the heels, 219;
see also breath; breathing exercises
breathing exercises, 72, 78, 102, 129, 142,
151–6, 167–70, 187, 189–90, 200, 215,
220; *see also* breathing; exercises; qi
gong

calm, 159, 164
central storehouse (Ren 12, zhong wan), 80
centre, 18, 21, 22, 48, 69, 70, 80, 102
centre of the chest (Ren 17, tan zhong),
80–1
chakras, 22, 52, 60, 117
chang qiang *see* long and strong
change, 13–14, 16, 17, 19, 35, 49, 54 108,
110, 160, 162, 164, 193
chest, 20, 40, 44, 47, 52, 64, 80, 91, 94, 102,
113, 116, 143, 152, 165, 187, 188, 190,
215, 220, 222
children, 214, 221, 222–3
Chinese angelica, 233
Chinese medicine, 5–6; history of, 3–4
chong mai *see* penetrating vessel
Chronic Fatigue Syndrome, 52–3, 171,
188, 219
circulation of light, 151–4, 207, 219
climate, 33
clouds, 160
cold, 15, 18, 20, 28, 40, 41, 44, 45, 74, 93,
170, 204, 224
colon, 20
colours, 16, 23, 38, 162
compassion, 46, 180
concentration, 39, 81, 97, 107, 108,
116–18, 124, 142, 144, 151, 154; on

lower abdomen, 116, 170, 207, 215, 216, 231
conception vessel (ren mai), 10, 76–82, 84, 87, 88, 91, 93, 116, 118, 151, 152, 219, 229
Confucianism, 3, 4, 5, 104
consciousness, 23, 50, 52, 99, 101
conservation, 26
constipation, 198, 227
contraction, 16, 17, 20, 40, 47, 193
coughs, 222
creative expression, 179–80, 196

da zhui see great hammer
dai mai see girdle vessel
dairy produce, 222–3
dampness, 18, 21, 33–4, 225, 238
dan tian, 9, 52, 75
dang gui see Chinese angelica
Dao, 9
Daoism, 3, 4, 5, 104, 151, 155
death, 47
depression, 19, 34, 37, 46, 111, 160, 178
desire, 104, 160
diaphragm, 73, 148
diarrhoea, 45, 96, 224, 227
diet, 5, 28, 31, 32, 33, 34, 98, 99, 194–5, 222, 230; see also food
digestive organs, 148
digestive problems, 35, 178, 180, 189, 223–7
downwards movement, 14, 16, 18
dreams, 35, 50, 52, 180
dryness, 18, 20
du mai see governor vessel

ears, 81, 131
earth, 13–14, 16, 21, 26, 46, 47, 48, 62, 80, 85, 88, 109, 118, 121; and the spleen, 30, 32, 193–200
eczema, 20, 103, 222
eight extraordinary meridians, 59, 68–93 219; and primary yin and yang, 69–87; and yin and yang qiao mai, 87–90; and yin and yang wei mai, 90–3; see also conception vessel; girdle vessel; governor vessel; penetrating vessel
Eight Treasure Tea, 233
elbows, 127, 135, 138
emotions, 3, 19, 20, 21, 25, 35, 38, 43–9, 55, 64, 94, 96, 104, 159–61, 181, 233
energy, 13, 14, 21–2, 26, 43, 49, 62, 193; depletion, 210–11; and three centres of transformation, 93–104; see also qi
essence (jing), 25–6, 45, 53, 75, 76, 78, 79, 99, 102
excess, 19, 34, 226
excitement, 19, 44, 159
exercise, 5, 6, 28, 39, 47, 68, 69, 73, 79, 81, 178; oriental, 108–10; see also exercises

exercises, 78, 107, 119–40; balancing left and right sides, 140–51; basic prone position, 143; for the eyes, 213; for the heart, 165–70; for the kidneys, 172–6; for the liver, 182–7, 226; for menstrual disorders, 229–30; standing warm-up, 229–30; see also breathing exercises; qi gong
extending meridian (Bladder 62, shen mai), 90
eyebrow centre, 75, 81, 97
eyes, 19, 20, 36, 38, 66, 81, 82, 90, 129, 186, 209, 211–14; see also vision

fainting, 75
fear, 21, 44–5, 48, 49, 96
feet, 110, 118, 119, 120–1, 123, 132, 171, 204, 210, 217
feng fu see storehouse of the wind
feng shui, 62
fertility, 27, 29, 97
finger pressure, 66
fingers, stretching, 108, 126–7
fingertips, 64, 113, 116, 117, 119, 126 175, 205, 238
fire, 18, 19–20, 28, 37–8, 72, 79, 97, 102, 117, 118, 165, 193, 238; and the heart, 23, 25, 159–61; and water, 16, 17, 21, 24, 26, 88, 90, 94, 96, 103, 214, 215, 237
fits, 19, 49
five directions, 18, 19, 20, 118
five elements, 3, 5, 6, 14, 18–21, 37, 42, 93, 118, 159–200, 238, 241; see also earth; fire; metal; water; wood
five internal organs, 21–41, 43, 93; see also heart; liver; lungs; kidneys; spleen
five tastes, 33, 99, 193–4
flesh, 31
flu, 40
fluids see liquids
food, 6, 21, 24, 25, 28, 31, 32, 33, 38, 41, 80, 81, 84, 94, 96, 97, 98–100, 193–5, 222, 224, 230, 236; see also diet; nourishment
forehead, soothing, 205
form, 78
forward bends, 220
four seasons, 14–17, 108, 118, 171–2, 240; ritual for, 162–5
freeflow, 19, 33, 43, 45, 233–4
fright, 48–9

gall-bladder, 19, 38, 64, 65, 85, 87, 94, 120, 124, 129, 140, 144, 183, 185–6, 208, 209, 213
gate of life (Du 4, ming men), 9, 28, 72–3, 79, 85, 97, 117
gate to the origin (Ren 4, guan yuan), 79, 85, 116, 126, 152, 175, 210–11, 227, 231, 237
genitals, 36–7, 88
ginger bath, 204
girdle vessel (dai mai), 9, 85–7, 93, 229, 234

governor vessel (du mai), 9, 69, 70–6, 79, 82, 84, 87, 88, 91, 93, 116, 117, 140, 150, 151, 204, 219
great hammer (Du 14, da zhui), 74, 117
grief, 20, 43, 47, 49, 188
groin, 69, 124
guan yuan *see* gate to the origin
gushing spring (Kidney 1, yong quan), 118, 123, 176

hair, 20, 27, 29, 41
hall of the seal (yin tang), 75
hands, 93, 113, 116, 126–7, 135, 165, 190–1
head, 75, 81, 82, 88, 91, 110, 117, 126, 131
headaches, 20, 34, 35, 36, 37, 38, 50, 74, 90, 110, 178, 180, 185, 203–11, 230, 233; and aggressive liver energy, 208–10; and energy depletion, 210–11; and eye strain, 211–14; and yin/yang imbalance, 203–8
healing, 165, 167
heart, 5–6, 19, 21, 22–5, 33, 43–4, 45, 76, 94, 99, 100, 117, 150, 188, 189, 194; acupuncture points, 73, 74; aversion to heat, 24; and blood vessels, 23; as emperor, 22; exercises for, 165–70; and fire element, 23, 25, 159; and insomnia, 215; and joy, 159–61; and kidneys, 24–5, 48; meridians, 64, 66, 116, 143, 165, 167; and small intestine, 25; and speech, 23–4; and the spirits, 22–3, 50, 51, 53; and upper burning space, 101–4; *see also* heart master
heart master, 64, 91, 102, 126, 165
heat, 14, 18, 19, 24, 38, 159, 204, 236, 238; *see also* fire
heaven, 13–14, 16, 26, 62, 76, 81, 82, 85, 101, 159, 160, 164
heavenly chimney (Ren 22, tian tu), 81–2
heavy periods, 235–6
heels, 87–8, 155, 219
herbal remedies, 4, 6, 33, 52, 99, 218, 222, 226, 233, 234–5, 237
hernia, 124
hips, 112, 123–4, 132, 142
hip-width apart, 190
hot flushes, 236, 237
humanity, 43, 46, 180
humility, 165, 169
hun, 9, 51, 179
hyperactivity, 23
hypertension, 164

I Ching, 69
ideas, 6, 53, 100, 101; *see also* intelligence; mind; thought
immunity, 97, 102
immunization, 222, 223
impotence, 29

incontinence, 79, 124
India, 52, 54, 60, 78, 119, 155, 167
infertility, 29, 79, 97
inner gateway (Heart Master 6, nei guan), 91
insomnia, 19, 22, 23, 48, 90, 94, 109, 159, 164, 214–16, 217, 219
intelligence, 26, 51, 52, 102
internal organs, 5–6, 19, 20, 21, 50, 151; *see also* five internal organs
intestines, 94, 227; *see also* large intestine; small intestine
inward movement, 14, 15, 18, 20
irritability, 34, 35, 50, 110, 233

Japan, 3–4, 17, 60, 61, 70, 73, 80, 97, 101, 104, 154, 161, 162, 170, 179, 181, 194
jing *see* essence
joints, 36, 176, 237, 238–9
joy, 19, 43–4, 49, 109, 159–61, 164
jue yin, 64
jumpiness, 48
justice, 43, 47

kidneys, 20, 21, 25–30, 32, 33, 34, 72, 94, 103, 116, 123, 148; and the bladder, 30; and bones and marrow, 27; and breathing problems, 221; concentration on, 117–18; exercises for, 172–6; and fear, 44–5; and the gate of life, 28; and the heart, 24–5, 48; and insomnia, 215, 216; and jing essence, 25–6; and the liver, 48–9; and lower burning space, 96–8; massage to, 172, 211, 223; meridian, 64, 79, 82, 88, 90, 112, 121, 124, 135, 204, 229; and reproduction, 29; and root of former heaven, 28; spirit of, 51, 53, 54; strengthening, 217–18; warming, 221
knees, 123, 132, 176, 200

large intestine, 20, 41, 64, 96–7, 126, 191, 227
legs, 62, 64, 79, 84, 88, 116, 123, 124, 144, 229
letting go, 41, 46, 110
leucorrhea, 45
life, 16, 17, 26, 34, 46, 62, 81
lifestyle, 110–11
ling tai *see* spirit watchtower
liquids, 27, 39, 78, 85, 96, 97, 98
little finger, 165, 167
liu wei di huang wan, 218, 237
liver, 19, 21, 29, 31, 33, 34–9, 48, 50, 81, 87, 94, 99, 208–10, 226, 233; and anger, 45–6, 208; and the blood, 35–6; and channel to genitals, 36–7; exercises for, 182–7; and the eyes, 38; and the

emotions, 43; and fire, 37–8; and freeflow, 34–5; and the gall-bladder, 38; meridian, 64, 66, 79, 110, 116, 121, 124, 185–6, 208, 229; and physical movement, 36; spirit of, 51–2; and the spleen, 195, 226; and wind, 36, 37; and wood element, 178–87
long and strong (Du 1, chang qiang), 72
loss, 47
lower abdomen, 20, 45, 54, 69, 70, 75, 76, 78, 79, 85, 87, 93, 94, 96, 102, 112, 113, 118, 124, 165, 170, 171, 175, 229, 230; breathing, 110, 218, 221; concentration on, 80, 116, 170, 207, 215, 216, 231, 237
lower burning space, 94, 96–8, 102
loyalty, 48
lungs, 20, 21, 33, 39–41, 64, 82, 94, 96, 99, 103, 116, 126, 143, 150, 221; aversion to the cold, 40; exercises to strengthen, 189–93, 220; and large intestine, 41; and metal element, 187–93; and the nose, 39–40; and qi, 39; and skin and body hair, 41; and sorrow, 46–7; spirit of, 50, 52–3; and the voice, 40

mania, 19, 23, 164
marrow, 27, 54
martial arts, 54, 97, 103, 120, 131, 178
massage, 4, 5, 6, 28, 47, 66, 81, 110, 238; abdominal, 198, 225, 227; bladder, 205; ears, 131; eyes, 129; feet, 123, 204, 210, 217; fingers, 127, 238; gall-bladder, 209; head, 131; kidneys, 172–6, 211, 223; large intestine, 227; liver, 210, 226; shoulders, 127, 209–10; spleen, 235–6; upper back, 223; see also self-massage
meditation, 23, 25, 27, 52, 68, 69, 70, 74, 75, 80, 81, 97, 109, 142, 154, 160, 164, 167, 169, 175, 207, 215, 237
men, 26, 29, 37, 70
Meng zi, 104
menopause, 24, 236–7
menstrual disorders, 35, 50, 84, 227–36
menstruation, 29, 36, 80, 124, 126, 196, 230; see also menstrual disorders
meridians, 6–7, 10, 59–61, 91, 116, 146, 151, 154, 165; exercises to stimulate qi in, 119–40; see also eight extraordinary meridians; 12 main meridians
metal, 16–17, 18, 20, 40, 41, 53, 96, 118; and the lungs, 187–93
middle burning space, 80, 94, 98–101
migraine, 34, 37, 38, 46, 178, 180, 195–6
mind, 23, 50, 93, 104, 181; calming the, 168–70, 214–16
ming men see gate of life
moon-gazing, 213
Morant, Soulie de, 4
Motoyama, Dr Hiroshi, 70, 100, 119
mouth, 33, 75–6, 82

movement, 14, 15, 36, 39, 47, 70, 78, 108, 110, 178, 183
moxa/moxibustion, 10, 73, 80, 210–11, 218, 221, 231, 238; for the spleen, 196, 198, 224, 235
muscles, 19, 31, 36, 37, 38, 48, 49, 72, 74, 93, 110, 210; relaxing, 216
music, 44

nausea, 208, 226
neck, 74, 81, 110, 117, 126, 129, 138, 140, 203, 205, 209
Nei Jing, 22, 29
neuropeptides, 101
night sweats, 217
nipples, 34, 66
nose, 39–40, 75–6, 81, 82
nostrils, alternate breathing through, 155–6
nourishment, 13, 21, 30, 31, 41, 62, 91; see also diet; food
numerology, 69, 82
nutrition see diet; food

obsession, 21, 195
one hundred meetings (Du 20, bai hui), 75, 117
oppression, 46, 49
original energy (yuan qi), 102
original essence, 102; see also essence (jing)
origins of life, 102
outer gateway (Triple Heater 5, wai guan), 91, 93
outward movement, 14, 15, 18, 19, 34, 35, 45, 46
overlooking tears (Gall–bladder 41, lin qi), 87

palace of impressions, 73
palms, 64, 117, 127, 165, 168, 175, 190, 211
palpitations, 19, 22, 48, 109, 159, 164, 194, 237
pathways, 61, 62–6, 68
penetrating vessel (chong mai), 9, 82–4, 87, 93, 102, 116, 229
pericardium see heart master
perineum, 37, 70, 72, 78, 79
period pains, 126, 230
ping chuan wan, 222
pituitary gland, 75
PMT, 185–6, 233–5; see also menstrual disorders; menstruation
po, 10, 52, 189
pores, 20, 41, 81, 93
posture, 40, 141
pregnancy, 49, 217, 226
premenstrual symptoms, 178, 208; see also PMT
psoriasis, 20
psyche, 30, 31

psychic powers, 53, 100, 101, 165, 167, 180
pulse, 188
purpose (yi), 53

qi, 21–2, 26, 29, 32, 33, 34, 35, 49, 53, 62, 81, 84, 93, 101, 154, 193; exercises to stimulate, 119–40; and the liver, 38; and the lungs, 39, 40; sea of, 79–80; see also energy
qi gong, 4, 6, 10, 68, 72, 75, 80, 103, 107 108, 109, 178, 219; balancing left and right sides, 150–1; balancing yin and yang, 236–7; basic pose, 112–19; for the heart, 165, 167; for the liver, 183, 185; for the lungs, 187, 189, 190–1; meditation, 175; movements, 113–16; simplified movements, 118–19; sitting position, 119; for the spleen and stomach, 200
qiao mai, 10, 87–90, 155, 207–8, 218–20

receivers, 100
relating, 180–2
relaxation, 107, 110, 143, 214, 216
Relaxed Wanderer, 226, 234–5
ren mai see conception vessel
repression, 19, 24, 37, 43, 160, 178
reproduction, 29
rest, 231
rhythm, 52, 53, 80, 88, 101, 167–8, 215, 220
ribcage, 87, 117, 168, 173, 183, 190, 198
ritual, 43, 44, 47, 161–5
root of former heaven, 28
root of later heaven, 28, 32
rotation, 21
routine, 216

sadness, 20, 46, 47, 49, 188
scientific medicine, 4, 5, 61
sea of liquid, 98
sea of qi (qi hai), 79–80, 116, 152, 175, 210–11, 221
self-healing, 3, 4
self-massage, 69, 107, 120; see also massage
sex, 26, 54, 94, 97, 98, 217
shao yang, 66
shao yin, 24, 64
shen (spirit), 26–7, 50, 51
shen dao see way of the spirits
shen mai see extending meridian
shiatsu massage, 4, 6
shining sea (Kidney 6, zhao hai), 88, 90
shock, 23, 66
shoulders, 47, 74, 117, 127, 138, 143, 190, 191, 203, 209–10
shoulder-width apart, 112, 131, 172, 182
side, 85, 140, 142, 182, 234

simplicity, 17
skin, 20, 41, 220
sleep, 35–6, 90, 189, 218–19; see also insomnia
small intestine, 25, 64, 65, 96, 126, 165, 227
sorrow, 46–7
soul see hun; po
spasms, 36, 38, 49, 93, 210
speech, 23–4
spine, 27, 54, 70, 72, 73, 74, 76, 117, 151, 152; stretches, 144–8; twists, 148–50, 186
spirit(s), 16, 19, 22–3, 36, 44, 49–54, 64, 73–4, 76, 94, 101, 102, 104, 150, 152, 159, 164; and the emotions, 55; and the heart, 22, 50, 51, 53; and the liver, 51–2; and the lungs, 50, 52–3; and the spleen, 51, 53; see also hun; shen
spirit watchtower (Du 10, ling tai), 73
spleen, 6, 21, 28, 30–4, 47–8, 80, 82, 94, 116; aversion to dampness, 33–4; and the blood, 31–2; and the earth, 30, 32, 193–200; and the liver, 195, 226; meridian, 64, 79, 121, 124, 229; and middle burning space, 98–101; and the mouth, 33; moxibustion for, 196, 198, 224, 235; and the muscles and flesh, 31; qi, 32, 33; and root of later heaven, 32; spirit of, 51, 53; and the stomach, 34; strengthening, 223–5; stretches for, 198, 200; and transformation, 30, 31; weakness of, 195, 235, 238
spring, 14, 16, 18, 19, 45, 46, 118, 162, 172, 178
standing qi gong, 165, 167
standing warm-up, 131–40
stillness, 17, 23, 94, 104, 107, 109, 163 164
stomach, 21, 28, 30, 31, 32, 34, 80, 82, 84, 94, 193, 196, 198, 211, 218, 224; meridian, 64–5, 120; and middle burning space, 98–101
storehouse of the wind (Du 16, feng fu), 74
stress, 154, 191, 193, 204
stretching exercises, 47, 108, 127, 129, 131, 138, 204, 234; for the kidneys, 172–3; for the liver, 182, 185–6; for lungs and large intestine, 191, 193; for the neck, 205, 209; spine, 140–8; for spleen and stomach, 198, 200
strokes, 38, 46
subtle energies, 59–61, 68, 151, 178
summer, 14, 16, 18, 19, 25, 40, 118, 162–3, 171, 193
sun-bathing, 213
surging qi (Stomach 30, qi chong), 84
swelling, 238
swimming, 189
symbolism, 3, 6, 69

tai ji, 75, 82, 103, 108, 131, 178
tai ji quan, 4, 10
tai yang, 66
tai yin, 64
tan zhong see centre of the chest
taste, sense of, 33, 99; see also five tastes
technology, medical, 2
teeth, 27, 29, 54, 75
television, watching, 214, 216
tendons, 19, 36
tension, 74, 142
thought, 20, 21, 27, 47–8, 74, 100, 214
three burning spaces, 94–104, 151
three centres of energy transformation, 93–104
three heaters see three burning spaces
Three Treasures, 26–7
throat, 90, 91
tiredness, 210
toes, 119, 120–1, 123
tongue, 23, 66, 75
toxins, 185
transformation, 6, 21, 26, 28, 30, 31, 32, 33, 37, 50, 70, 72, 76, 93–104, 193, 225
transmitters, 100
trembling, 36, 37
triple heater, 64, 91, 93, 102, 126, 129, 165, 213
truth, 43, 48
12 main meridians, 39, 59, 62–7, 68, 84, 93; triple heater, 64; yang, 62, 65–6; yin, 62, 64

uniting heaven and earth, 200
upper abdomen, 80, 94, 152
upper burning space, 94, 100, 101–4, 188
upper sea of qi, 80, 102
upwards movement, 14, 16, 18, 19, 34, 35, 37, 43, 45, 46, 87, 159

vaginal discharges, 85
vertigo, 37
violence, 17, 34, 45, 46
'virtues', 43, 44, 45, 46, 47, 48, 161
vision, 37, 38, 208
visualisation, 68, 69, 70, 74, 79, 165, 167, 170, 219, 238
voice, 40
vomiting, 226

waist, 85, 132, 135, 148, 183
waking, 217
walking, 47, 121, 178, 186–7, 189, 207, 210, 216, 220, 234
warmth, 170–1, 221, 223, 224, 231
water, 16, 17, 18, 20–1, 24, 26, 45, 78, 88, 90, 94, 103, 118, 193, 214, 237; and kidneys, 27, 170–6
way of the spirits (Du 11, shen dao), 73–4

wei mai, 10, 90–3
weight gain or loss, 224
will (zhi), 53, 54
wind, 18, 19, 35, 41, 45, 69, 74, 93, 103, 119, 178; and the liver, 36, 37, 38
windows of heaven, 81
winter, 14, 16, 17, 18, 20, 25, 40, 44, 118, 162, 163–4, 170, 171, 172
wisdom, 43, 44, 45, 98
women, 26, 29, 36, 49, 70, 80, 85, 179, 217, 227–36; see also menopause; menstrual disorders; menstruation; PMT; pregnancy
Women's Precious formula, 233, 235
wood, 16–17, 18, 19, 34, 36, 37, 38, 45, 46, 118, 121, 178–87, 193, 208, 210
worry, 21, 47
wrists, 119, 126–7, 135, 238

xiao yao wan see Relaxed Wanderer

yang, 3, 5, 10, 24, 26, 27, 34, 35, 36, 45, 49, 78, 82, 84, 117, 118, 143, 154, 159, 187, 195, 240; balance with yin, 87–8, 203–8, 214, 236–7; and elements, 19; and four seasons, 14–17; and headaches, 203–4; and heaven, 13–14, 62; and the kidneys, 54; and the liver, 37, 38; meridians, 59, 64, 65–6, 91, 111, 112, 121, 126; original, 93; pathways, 62, 76; primary, 69–87; qiao mai, 87–90, 155, 207–8, 218–20; wei mai, 90–3
yang ming, 66
yang qi see breath
yellow emperor (Spleen 4, gong sun), 84
Yellow Emperor's Classic of Internal Medicine, The, 22, 29, 50, 96, 171–2
yi see purpose
yin, 3, 5, 10, 24, 26, 35, 36, 45, 49, 53, 76, 78, 82, 84, 150, 154, 240; balance with yang, 87–8, 203–8, 214, 236–7; and the earth, 13–14, 62; essence, 29; and four seasons, 14–17, 164; and kidneys, 54; and liver, 37, 38, 51, 52; meridians, 59, 64, 91, 111, 112, 116, 118, 121, 126, 143, 229; original, 93; pathways, 62; primary, 69–87; qiao mai, 87–90, 155, 207–8, 218–20; wei mai, 90–3
yin crossing, 75–6
yin meeting, 78–9
yin tang see hall of the seal
yoga, 54, 81, 119, 140, 155, 167, 178, 189
yong quan see gushing spring

zhi see will
Zhuang zi, 104
zong qi see ancestral qi